INTRODUCTION TO VETERINARY ANATOMY AND Physiology WORKBOOK

Commissioning Editors: Rita Demetriou-Swanwick, Robert Edwards
Development Editor: Louisa Welch
Project Manager: Andrew Palfreyman
Designer/Design Direction: Stewart Larking
Illustrations Manager: Merlyn Harvey

SECOND EDITION

INTRODUCTION TO VETERINARY ANATOMY AND Physiology WORKBOOK

Sally Bowden BSc(Hons) CertEd RVN

Past senior examiner and assessor for the RCVS and ABC
Examiner and lecturer in veterinary nursing and animal care
Christchurch, New Zealand

BUTTERWORTH HEINEMANN

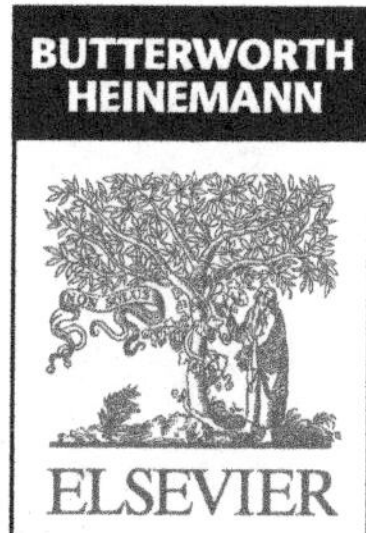

ELSEVIER

Edinburgh London New York Oxford Philadelphia St Louis Sydney Toronto 2009

BUTTERWORTH
HEINEMANN
ELSEVIER

An Imprint of Elsevier Ltd.

First published 2003
This edition 2009

ISBN 978-0-7020-5232-3

British Library Cataloguing in Publication Data
A catalogue record for this book is available from the British Library

Library of Congress Cataloging in Publication Data
A catalog record for this book is available from the Library of Congress

Notice
Knowledge and best practice in this field are constantly changing. As new research and experience broaden our knowledge, changes in practice, treatment and drug therapy may become necessary or appropriate. Readers are advised to check the most current information provided (i) on procedures featured or (ii) by the manufacturer of each product to be administered, to verify the recommended dose or formula, the method and duration of administration, and contraindications. It is the responsibility of the practitioner, relying on their own experience and knowledge of the patient, to make diagnoses, to determine dosages and the best treatment for each individual patient, and to take all appropriate safety precautions. To the fullest extent of the law, neither the Publisher nor the Editor assumes any liability for any injury and/or damage to persons or property arising out of or related to any use of the material contained in this book.

Neither the Publisher nor the Editor assumes any responsibility for any loss or injury and/or damage to persons or property arising out of or related to any use of the material contained in this book. It is the responsibility of the treating practitioner, relying on independent expertise and knowledge of the patient, to determine the best treatment and method of application for the patient.

The Publisher

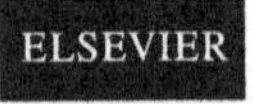

Transferred to Digital Printing in 2012

Contents

CHAPTER 1

Body composition and cells

LEARNING Objectives

This chapter will help you revise the following:
- facts about body composition
- body water
- atoms, ions and electrolytes
- homeostatic mechanisms
- metabolism
- facts about cells
- the general structure and function of the animal cell
- cellular processes
- cell division.

There is a general revision section at the end of the chapter.

Facts about body composition

1. The animal body is made up of both inorganic and organic substances.
2. The inorganic components of the body are:
   a. water
   b. minerals.
3. The organic components of the body are:
   a. cells
   b. miscellaneous fibres and membranes (see Ch. 2, 'Body Tissues and Cavities', for more information).

Look it up

Exercise 1.1 We hear the word organic mentioned a lot but what exactly does it mean? Likewise, what does inorganic mean? Look up these words in the dictionary and write their definitions below:

(1)Organic: ____

(2)Inorganic: ____

Body water

Key Points:

1. water is a key constituent of the animal body and is essential for life
2. water has many functions in the animal body, including the following:
   a. it is a medium in which substances are dissolved or suspended
   b. it is essential in order for many chemical reactions to occur
   c. it provides transport for nutrients
   d. it facilitates removal of toxins and wastes from the body
   e. it is the main constituent of many secretions, e.g. saliva.

Fill in the gaps

Exercise 1.2 Complete the paragraph by filling in the gaps using the correct words from the selection below.

- cutaneous
- interstitial
- compartments
- higher
- lacrimation
- intracellular
- 60–70
- respiratory
- urinary
- obese
- extracellular
- insensible
- gastrointestinal
- lower
- intravascular

Water makes up (1)__________% of the body, although this figure may be (2)__________ in a young animal and (3)__________ in an elderly or (4)__________ animal. Water is found in many different areas of the body, often referred to as body (5)__________.

The two main body compartments are the area inside the cells and the area outside the cells. The water found inside the cells is called (6)__________ fluid or ICF—this is where two-thirds of body water is situated. The area outside the cells is called (7)__________ fluid or ECF. The extracellular body compartment is then divided further in three areas:

- the fluid in between the body tissues, in the tissue spaces, known as (8)__________ fluid
- the fluid in the blood and lymphatic vascular systems, known as (9)__________ fluid
- the fluid in the body cavities and tracts, known as transcellular fluid.

Water moves between the body compartments by osmosis but is also constantly being lost from the body via several routes:

- (10)__________ tract—evaporation during breathing
- (11)(__________)—evaporation during sweating
- (12)__________ tract—in faeces and vomit
- urinary tract—in urine.

There are other minor routes, such as vaginal discharge and (13)__________. It is vital that each body compartment is correctly hydrated, so the animal must replace what is lost by eating and drinking sufficient water each day. The body can control water loss by the (14)__________ and gastrointestinal routes to some degree. However, it cannot control losses by the respiratory and cutaneous routes—these losses are sometimes termed inevitable or (15)__________.

Activity

Exercise 1.3 Complete the table below by writing the correct amount of water lost via each route per 24 hours.

Route	Amount in ml per kg per 24 hours
Breathing	(1)
Sweating	(2)
Faeces	(3)
Urine	(4)
Total	(5)

Atoms, ions and electrolytes

Key Points:

1. The body contains minerals in the form of ions.
2. Examples of minerals found in the body are calcium, phosphorus, potassium and sodium.
3. *Ions* are atoms with a charge.
4. Atoms are structures with a nucleus of neutrons and positively charged protons with one or more outer 'shells' containing negatively charged electrons.
5. When the number of electrons (−ve) exceeds the number of protons (+ve), the ion is negatively charged and is known as an *anion*.
6. When the number of protons (+ve) exceeds the number of electrons (−ve), the ion is positively charged and is known as a *cation*.
7. A substance that breaks down into ions when dissolved in water is called an *electrolyte*.

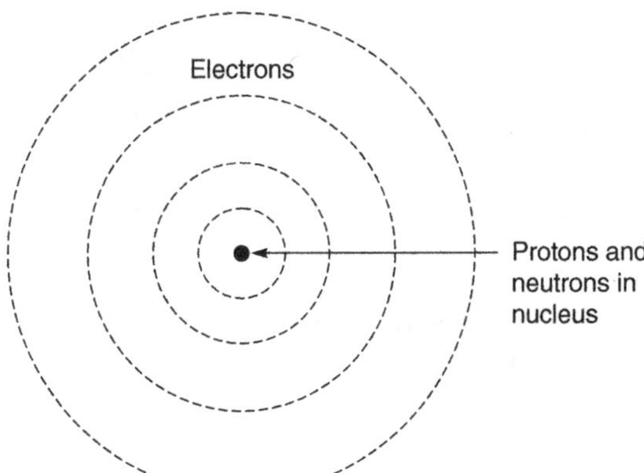

Figure 1.1 Diagram of an atom.
(Reproduced with kind permission from Bowden & Masters 2001.)

Link the words

Exercise 1.4 Match the descriptions in the left-hand column to the definitions in the right-hand column by drawing a line to link them.

(1)Minerals are	(2)atoms with a positive charge
(3)Ions are	(4)atoms with a negative charge
(5)Cations are	(6)substances which break down into ions when dissolved in water
(7)Anions are	(8)atoms with a charge
(9)Electrolytes are	(10)found in the body in the form of ions

Activity

Exercise 1.5 Complete the table below to show the chemical symbol of the following ions and whether they are cations or anions.

Ion	Symbol	+ or –?
Sodium	(1)	(2)
Chlorine	(3)	(4)
Potassium	(5)	(6)
Calcium	(7)	(8)
Phosphorus	(9)	(10)
Magnesium	(11)	(12)

Homeostatic mechanisms

Key Points:

1. Homeostasis is the name for the maintenance of optimal conditions in which the body functions at its best.
2. There are many homeostatic mechanisms, such as:
   a. osmoregulation—maintenance of optimal fluid levels in all body compartments
   b. thermoregulation—maintenance of optimal body temperature
   c. excretion of waste products to prevent toxic build-up
   d. buffer systems—maintenance of the correct pH
   e. blood pressure maintenance
   f. correct metabolic rate.
3. Many of these mechanisms are a function of the kidney (see Ch. 10, 'Urinary System', for more information).
4. Maintenance of homeostasis is also reliant on feedback from other body systems to give information, i.e. the endocrine system or the nervous system.

Activity

Exercise 1.6 Complete the table below to show the parameters of an animal maintaining homeostasis.

Measurement	Dog	Cat
Body temperature	(1)	(2)
pH of body fluids	(3)	(4)
Urine output	(5)	(6)

(Continued)

Specific gravity of urine	(7)	(8)
Fluid intake	(9)	(10)
Blood pressure	(11)	(12)

Metabolism

Key Points:

1. The metabolism is the sum total of the chemical reactions taking place in the body.
2. There are different types of chemical reaction:
   a. anabolic reactions, which build simple substances into complex ones with the use of energy
   b. catabolic reactions, which break complex substances into simple ones with the release of energy.
3. The substances taking part in these reactions are called metabolites and are obtained from food.
4. The metabolic rate of an animal (when it is at rest, not stressed or ill and is not in a particularly hot or cold environment) is known as the basal metabolic rate, i.e. BMR.

Facts about cells

1. The cell is the smallest individually functioning unit of the animal body.
2. Cells are microscopic—their size varies but averages around 0.02 mm in diameter.
3. Cells will only live for a certain length of time, after which they die and break down.
4. Cells are constantly dying and being replaced throughout an animal's life.
5. Body tissue is made up of a group of cells performing a specialized function or functions.
6. A body organ is a group of body tissues performing a specialized function or functions.
7. The prefix denoting a cell is *cyt–*.

List the structures

Look at some cells using a microscope. These may be from a vaginal smear, urine sample or other part of the body. Make a note of the cells' appearance. What structures can you see?

General structure and function of a cell

Key Points:

1. There are many different types of cell that perform a variety of functions but most have a similar structure.
2. The parts of a cell necessary for it to function are called the organelles.
3. Other structures sometimes found in cells are called inclusion bodies. These may be normal, such as the pigment melanin, or disease-induced, such as Negri bodies seen in animals that have contracted rabies.

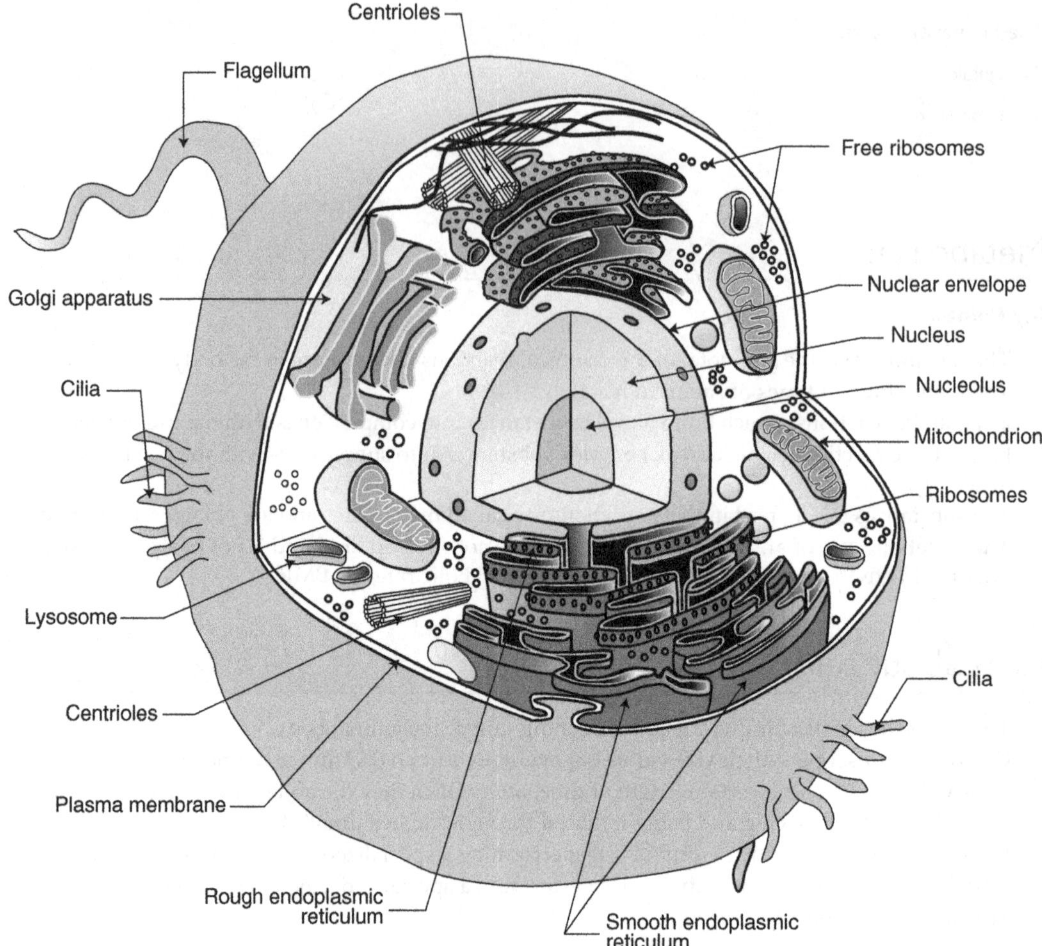

Figure 1.2 Diagram of a mammalian cell.
(Reproduced with kind permission from Colville & Bassert 2002.)

Link the words

Exercise 1.7 Match the description in the left-hand column to the correct definition in the right-hand column by drawing a line to link them.

(1)Made up of two centrioles, concerned with cell reproduction	(2)Cell membrane
(3)A space in the cytoplasm, often caused by engulfed particles	(4)Mitochondria
(5)The outer lining of the cell, which is semipermeable. Substances are transported across by a number of methods	(6)Centrosome

(Continued)

(7)Membranes responsible for surrounding and removing harmful material from the cell	(8)Golgi complex
(9)Tubes that store substances, e.g. lysosomal enzymes	(10)Nucleus
(11)Rough – the site of protein synthesis by ribosomes. Smooth – the site of lipid synthesis	(12)Lysosomes
(13)Jelly-like substance that gives the cell its shape. Contains nucleus and other substances such as glucose and salts	(14)Endoplasmic reticulum
(15)Membranes responsible for energy release in the cell	(16)Cytoplasm
(17)Contains chromosomes that carry genetic information and a nucleolus that manufactures ribosomes. Absent in mature erythrocytes	(18)Vacuole

Cellular processes

Key Points:

1. Many processes take place inside a cell in order for it to function. As individually functioning units, each one needs to be able to obtain energy, expel waste, respire and reproduce.
2. In order for the cell to maintain optimal conditions and carry out its intended functions, substances must constantly cross the cell membrane or move into or out of the cell by other means. There are several ways in which this can occur:
   a. ***passive transport mechanisms*** (those that do not require energy):
      i. *osmosis* (the passage of water from a solution of low concentration to a solution of high concentration through the semipermeable membrane)
      ii. *diffusion* (the passage of solutes—particles dissolved in fluid—from a solution of high concentration to a solution of low concentration through the semipermeable membrane)
      iii. *facilitated transport* (solutes combine with a carrier molecule in the cell membrane)
   b. ***active transport mechanisms*** (those that require energy to occur):
      i. *membrane pumps*—these usually work in the absence of a favourable pressure gradient, i.e. the solution receiving the solute is more concentrated than the solution losing the solute (e.g. the sodium and potassium pump, which maintains a higher sodium content in ECF and a higher potassium content in ICF)
   c. endocytosis (uptake of material into the cell by invagination of the cell membrane). This occurs with hormones, immunoglobulins and foreign matter such as viruses. The taking in of solid matter is termed phagocytosis and the taking in of liquid matter is termed pinocytosis
   d. exocytosis (expelling matter from the cell by exvagination of the cell membrane). This occurs with neurotransmitter substances and hormones.

Fill in the gaps

Exercise 1.8 Complete the paragraph by filling in the gaps using the correct words from the selection below.

- concentrated
- less
- gradient
- water
- hypertonic
- diffusion
- higher
- equalize
- hypotonic
- isotonic
- membranes
- more

A semipermeable membrane is one that lets small molecules through but not large ones (imagine a mesh or sieve). Cell (1)____________ are semipermeable.

If there is a solution either side of the semipermeable membrane and one solution contains more molecules than the other, the side with more molecules is said to be more (2)____________ than the other. It is a law of physics that solutions will always try to (3)____________ in concentration site so if the molecules are small enough they will move across the semipermeable membrane from the more concentrated side to the less concentrated side until they have the same concentration. This is called (4)____________.

Another way for the solutions to equalize in concentration would be for the (5)____________ to move across the semipermeable membrane, from the (6)____________ concentrated side to the (7)____________ concentrated side until they have the same concentration. This is osmosis.

Osmotic pressure is a measure of how concentrated a solution is, i.e. the more concentrated a solution, the (8)____________ its osmotic pressure. The difference between the concentrations of two solutions is called the pressure (9)____________. A solution with the same osmotic pressure as the substance to which it is being compared is said to be (10)____________. A solution with a higher osmotic pressure than the substance to which it is being compared is said to be (11)____________. A solution with a lower osmotic pressure than the substance to which it is being compared is said to be (12)____________.

Cell division

Key Points:

1. Mitosis is the process by which all of the body's cells reproduce, except for the gametes. The end result is two identical daughter cells, each with the same number of chromosomes in their nuclei as the parent cell. This is called the diploid number.
2. Meiosis is the process by which the gametes are produced. It occurs in the gonads. The end result is four daughter cells each with half the number of chromosomes in their nuclei of the parent cell. This is called the haploid number and occurs so that when the male and female gametes (sperm and ovum) fuse at conception, the correct number of chromosomes for that species is restored.
3. Mitosis involves one round of cell division and meiosis involves two rounds of cell division.
4. During meiosis, the swapping of genetic information between chromosomes occurs. This is called 'crossing over'.
5. As meiosis results in a haploid number of chromosomes for each daughter cell, it is sometimes called 'reduction division'.
6. Of the four daughter cells resulting from meiosis in the female, only one will become an ovum. The other three structures become non-functional polar bodies.

Mnemonic

To differentiate mitosis and meiosis, remember this rhyme:

Mitosis occurs in **my** **t**oes
Meiosis occurs in **my** **o**varies

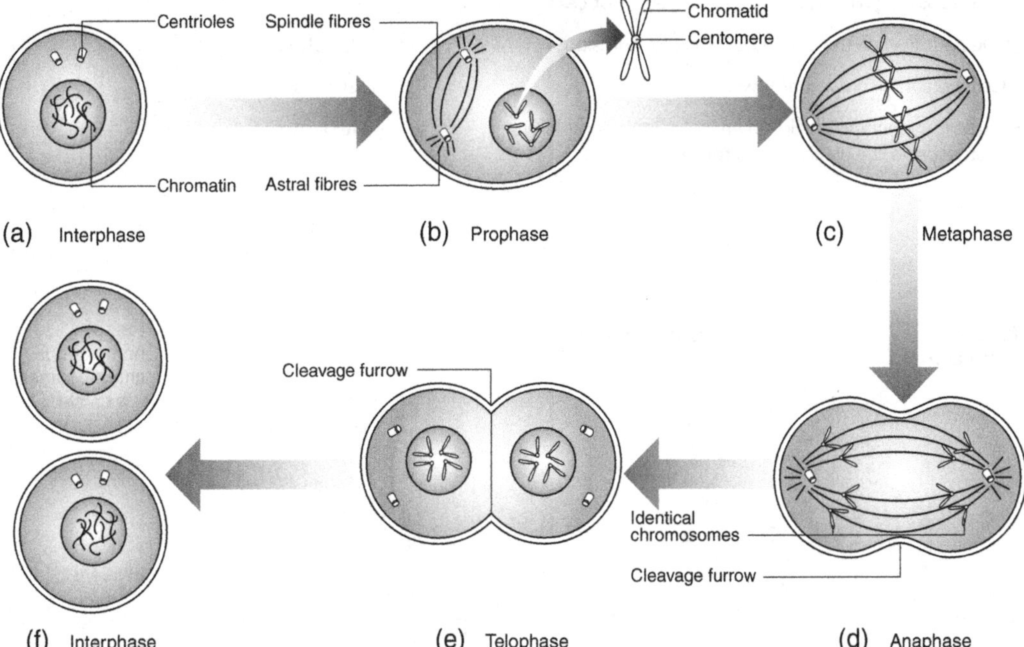

Figure 1.3 The stages of mitosis. (a) Interphase: before a cell can divide, it must first make a copy of its DNA and another pair of centromeres. (b) Prophase: chromatin strands coil and condense to form chromosomes, which are linked at a central kinetophore. A spindle apparatus takes form while the nuclear envelope disintegrates. (c) Metaphase: chromosomes line up in the centre of the spindle. The centromere of each chromosome is attached to a spindle fibre. (d) Anaphase: chromatids are pulled apart by spindle fibres to form a duplicate set of chromosomes. The cytoplasm constricts at the metaphyseal plate. (e) Telophase: chromatin begins to unravel at the poles of the cell and a nuclear envelope appears. Cytokinesis marks the end of telophase. (f) Interphase: the cycle of growth is repeated.
(Adapted from Colville & Bassert 2002.)

Mnemonic

To remember the phases of mitosis:

I paid **m**y **a**unt **t**wice!
Interphase
Prophase
Metaphase
Anaphase
Telophase

Link the words

Exercise 1.9 Match the description in the left-hand column to the correct definition in the right-hand column by drawing a line to link them.

(1)Chromosomes become visible in the nucleus	(2)Interphase
(3)Chromosomes separate into two chromatids. Chromatids are pulled apart to opposite edges of cell	(4)Prophase
(5)The period when the cell is not undergoing division	(6)Metaphase
(7)Cell membrane divides into two	(8)Anaphase
(9)Nuclear membrane breaks down and spindle fibres form. Chromosomes line up along equator of cell	(10)Telophase

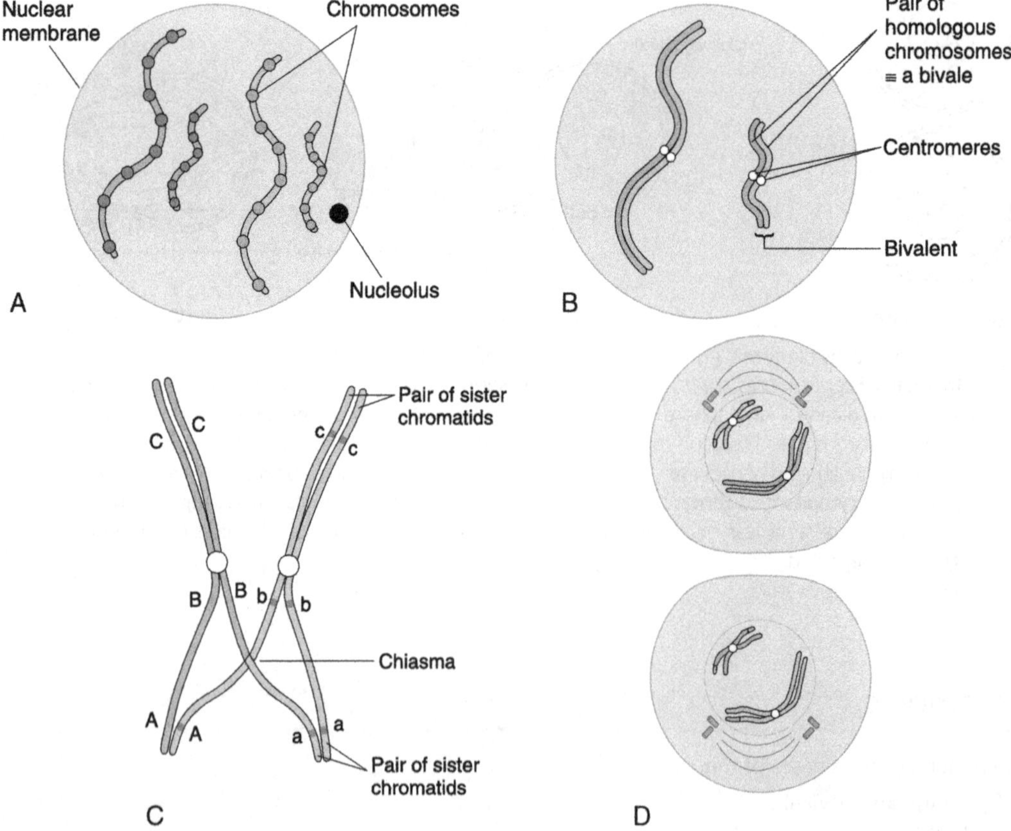

Figure 1.4 The stages of meiosis.
(Reproduced with kind permission from CAW et al 2005.)

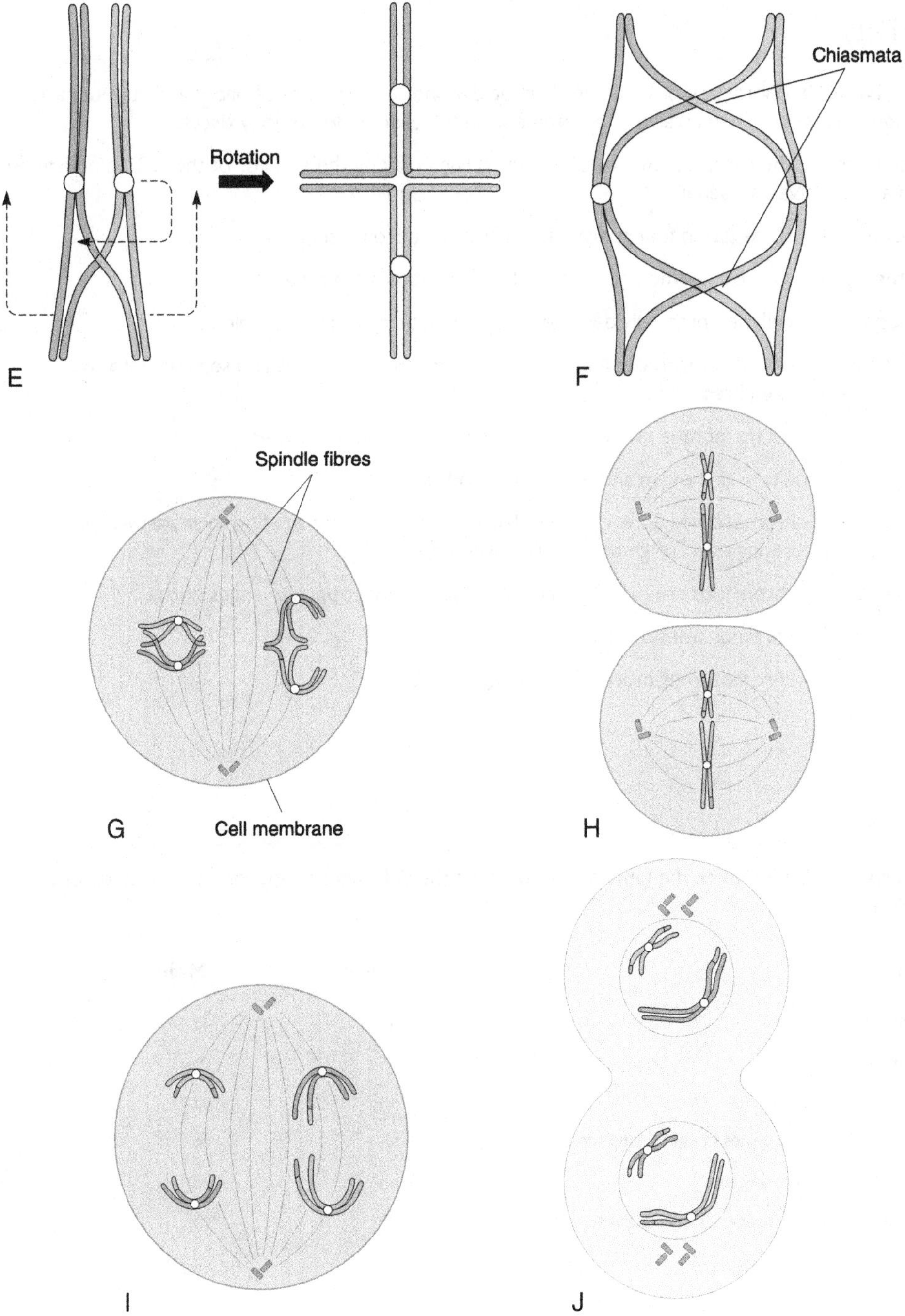

Figure 1.4 (Continued)

Activity

Exercise 1.10 Photocopy or copy the chart below onto a large piece of paper and cut out each individual sentence. Then arrange the statements in the order in which they occur.

(1)Metaphase I – the chromosome pairs (bivalents) line up along the equator of the cell. Spindle fibres form and the bivalents separate.

(2)Spermatogenesis results in four spermatids, which will become sperm.

(3)In the diploid germ cell, homologous pairs of chromosomes are separate.

(4)Telophase II – cell membrane divides; the second meiotic division is complete.

(5)Metaphase II – the chromosomes line up along the equator of the cell and separate into two chromatids. Spindle fibres form.

(6)Telophase I – cell membrane divides; the first meiotic division is complete.

(7)Oogenesis results in one ovum and three polar bodies.

(8)Prophase I – chromosomes double up and thicken. Homologous pairs find their partner (forming a bivalent) and 'crossing over' of genetic information occurs.

(9)Anaphase II – chromatids are pulled apart and move towards opposite edges of the cell.

(10)Prophase II – chromosomes thicken once again.

(11)Anaphase I – chromosomes move to the edge of the cell.

Activity

Exercise 1.11 Complete the table below to depict the differences between the two types of cell division.

Feature	**Mitosis**	**Meiosis**
Site in body	(1)	(2)
Rounds of division	(3)	(4)
Number of daughter cells	(5)	(6)
Number of chromosomes in each daughter cell	(7)	(8)
Occurrence of 'crossing over'	(9)	(10)
Appearance of daughter cells in relation to each other	(11)	(12)

Activity

Design a poster on A3 paper depicting the different stages of mitosis and meiosis. Use large labels and bold colours. When it is complete, stick it up somewhere you will regularly read it. Why not on a kitchen cupboard?

General revision

Multiple choice questions – body composition

Exercise 1.12

1. An organic substance is one that:
   a. contains chemical fertilizer
   b. contains carbon
   c. may be burnt on site
   d. may be disposed of in general waste.
2. The routes of fluid loss termed insensible are:
   a. faecal and urinary
   b. respiratory and urinary
   c. cutaneous and respiratory
   d. urinary and cutaneous.
3. The amount of fluid lost via the urinary route per kg every 24 hours is approximately:
   a. 2 ml
   b. 20 ml
   c. 200 ml
   d. 2000 ml.
4. Body fluid has a pH of:
   a. 1.4
   b. 5.4
   c. 7.4
   d. 9.4.
5. A substance that breaks into ions when dissolved in water is a:
   a. cation
   b. anion
   c. electrolyte
   d. metabolite.
6. One of the main homeostatic organs is the:
   a. heart
   b. spleen
   c. stomach
   d. kidney.
7. The chemical symbol for potassium is:
   a. Na
   b. K
   c. Ca
   d. P.
8. A catabolic reaction:
   a. releases energy
   b. stores energy
   c. uses energy
   d. destroys energy.

Tip: *Why not get together with fellow students and write some more questions for each other?*

Word Chart

Exercise 1.13

1	B
2	O
3	D
4	Y
5	C
6	O
7	M
8	P
9	O
10	S
11	I
12	T
13	I
14	O
15	N

Clues

1. A body cavity where transcellular fluid could be found.
2. Minerals and water are this type of substance.
3. The condition where body pH is too low.
4. pH stands for 'per ________'.
5. The smallest individually functioning units of the animal body.
6. The percentage of the body made up of ICF.
7. Magnesium and potassium are both this.
8. The unit of measurement used to determine how acid or alkaline a substance is.
9. A process by which water moves across a semipermeable membrane.
10. The mineral Na.
11. A route of fluid loss, excreted by the kidney.
12. Another term for outside of the cells.
13. The mineral Ca.
14. Plasma is the fluid component of this substance.
15. This is an atom with a charge.

Tip: *Have you seen a word you don't understand? Don't ignore it—look it up!*

Multiple choice questions – cells

Exercise 1.14

1. The average diameter of a cell is:
   a. 0.02 mm
   b. 0.2 mm
   c. 2 mm
   d. 20 mm.
2. The only living cell in the canine and feline body with no nucleus is the:
   a. lymphocyte
   b. erythrocyte
   c. thrombocyte
   d. monocyte.
3. The cellular structures that can usually be seen using a compound microscope are:
   a. the nucleus, Golgi body and cell membrane
   b. the mitochondria, cytoplasm, ribosomes and vacuoles
   c. the nucleus, cytoplasm, vacuoles and cell membrane
   d. the ribosomes, Golgi body and nucleus.
4. Mitochondria are responsible for:
   a. surrounding and removing harmful material
   b. storing lysosomal enzymes
   c. energy release
   d. cell defence.
5. Genetic information is found in the form of:
   a. DNA
   b. lipid chains
   c. RNA
   d. glucose chains.
6. Endocytosis is:
   a. the passage of fluid through the semipermeable membrane
   b. exvagination of the cell membrane to expel matter from the cell
   c. the passage of molecules through the semipermeable membrane
   d. invagination of the cell membrane to take matter into the cell.
7. Active transport mechanisms:
   a. require energy
   b. do not require energy
   c. produce energy
   d. transport energy.
8. An example of a membrane pump is:
   a. the calcium and protein pump
   b. the phospholipid pump
   c. the sodium and potassium pump
   d. the cytoplasm pump.
9. If a cell is placed in a hypertonic solution it will:
   a. shrivel
   b. stay the same
   c. expand
   d. lyse

10. If a cell was placed in a concentrated chloride solution, chloride would:
    a. enter the cell by diffusion
    b. enter the cell by osmosis
    c. leave the cell by diffusion
    d. leave the cell by osmosis.
11. Mitosis occurs in:
    a. all body cells including the gonads
    b. all body cells except the gonads
    c. the male gonads only
    d. the gonads only.
12. Meiosis results in:
    a. two daughter cells with a diploid number of chromosomes
    b. two daughter cells with a haploid number of chromosomes
    c. four daughter cells with a diploid number of chromosomes
    d. four daughter cells with a haploid number of chromosomes.
13. The phase of mitosis when the spindle fibres form is:
    a. anaphase
    b. telophase
    c. prophase
    d. metaphase.
14. The phase of mitosis when the cell membrane divides is:
    a. interphase
    b. metaphase
    c. telophase
    d. anaphase.
15. The phase of meiosis when 'crossing over' occurs is:
    a. prophase I
    b. metaphase I
    c. prophase II
    d. metaphase II.

Tip: *Why not get together with fellow students and write some more questions for each other?*

Word Chart

Exercise 1.15

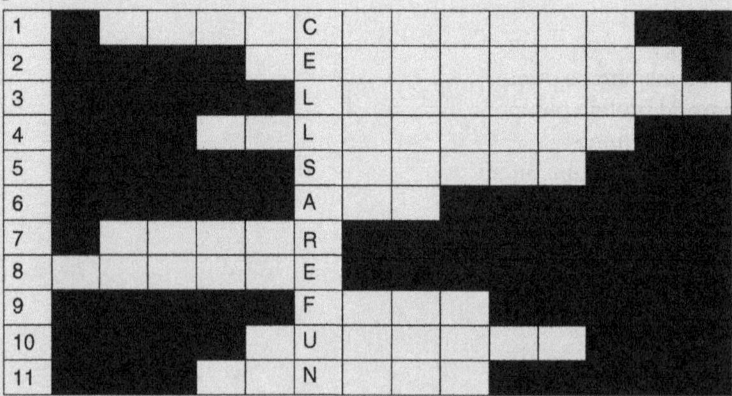

Clues

1. Taking in matter by invagination of the cell membrane.
2. Meiosis is sometimes called this type of division.
3. Membranes responsible for surrounding and removing harmful material from the cell.
4. The last phase of mitosis.
5. A membrane pump is constantly pumping this out of the cell.
6. Initials of the form of energy that is used in the body.
7. Oogenesis results in three of these bodies.
8. A transport mechanism that requires energy.
9. The number of spermatids resulting from spermatogenesis.
10. The control centre of the cell.
11. Where meiosis occurs.

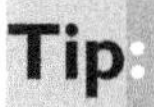

Have you seen a word you don't understand? Don't ignore it—look it up!

Activity

Prepare a five-minute presentation entitled 'Osmosis and Diffusion'. Your audience could be friends, family or fellow students. When you have finished, invite questions from the floor!

CHAPTER 2

Body tissues and cavities

LEARNING Objectives

This chapter will help you to revise the following:

- facts about and functions of body tissues
- epithelial tissue
- connective tissue
- muscle tissue (see Ch. 4, 'The Muscular System', for more information)
- nerve tissue (see Ch. 5, 'The Nervous System and Special Senses', for more information)
- facts about body cavities
- the thoracic cavity
- the abdominal cavity.

There is a general revision section at the end of the chapter.

Facts about and functions of body tissues

1. A tissue is a group of cells specialized to perform a function or functions.
2. Several tissues grouped together form an organ.
3. There are four main types of body tissue:
   a. muscle
   b. nerve
   c. epithelial tissue
   d. connective tissue.
4. All other body tissues fall into one of these four categories.

Mnemonic

To remember the four types of body tissue:

Mum **n**ever **e**ats **c**ake

Muscle
Nerve
Epithelial
Connective

Epithelial tissue

Key Points:

1. Epithelial tissue lines and covers surfaces.
2. There are two main types of epithelial tissue:
   a. simple
   b. compound.
3. All glands are made of epithelial tissue.
4. Mucous membrane is epithelial tissue that produces thick mucus to protect underlying tissues.
5. Serous membrane is epithelial tissue that produces a watery fluid to prevent friction, e.g. the body cavities.
6. In most places in the body epithelial tissue is called *epithelium* but the lining of the heart, blood vessels and lymph vessels is sometimes termed *endothelium*.

Fill in the gaps

Exercise 2.1 Complete the paragraphs below by filling in the gaps using the correct words from the selection below.

- foot pads
- reduced
- keratin
- cilia
- basement
- genital
- alveoli
- ureters
- urine
- liver
- oviduct
- goblet

Simple epithelial tissue

Simple epithelial tissues are those that are only one cell layer thick on a (1)__________ membrane. There are three main types of simple epithelial tissue—simple squamous, cuboidal and columnar. Simple squamous epithelial tissue is the finest, thinnest lining and is found in areas where it is important that there is no friction as well as where substances may need to pass through the tissue wall. Examples of where this is found are the blood vessel walls and the (2)__________. Cuboidal, or cubical epithelial tissue, is a specialized tissue found in the kidney tubules and the (3)__________. Columnar epithelial tissue often has small hairs or (4)__________ lining its free surface; it is then called ciliated columnar epithelial tissue. Often, single-celled glands in the tissue, called (5)__________ cells, produce mucus, which is moved along by the cilia. This 'conveyor belt' system is useful in places such as the nasal cavity, where the cilia and mucus move foreign matter away from the lower respiratory tract. It is also found in the (6)__________, where it aids the movement of ova, and in the digestive tract.

Compound epithelial tissue

Compound epithelial tissues are those that are more than one-cell-layer thick on a basement membrane. There are two main types of compound epithelial tissue—stratified squamous and transitional. Stratified squamous epithelial tissue is found in areas that are subject to trauma, such as the oral cavity and (7)__________ passage. The skin is also stratified squamous epithelial tissue but it has been infiltrated by a tough protein called (8)__________, which is why it has a different appearance. Different areas of the skin are more keratinized than others, e.g. the (9)__________.

Transitional epithelial tissue is found in the (10)__________, bladder and urethra. It has the ability to expand greatly, which is useful as the bladder fills with (11)__________. When this happens the number of cell layers is greatly (12)__________.

Activity

Exercise 2.2 All glands are made from epithelial tissue and produce a secretion. The prefix denoting a gland is *aden–*. There are two main types of gland—exocrine and endocrine. Fill in the chart below to show the differences between these two types of gland.

	Exocrine	Endocrine
General name for secretions	(1)	(2)
Method of reaching site of action	(3)	(4)
Proximity to site of action	(5)	(6)

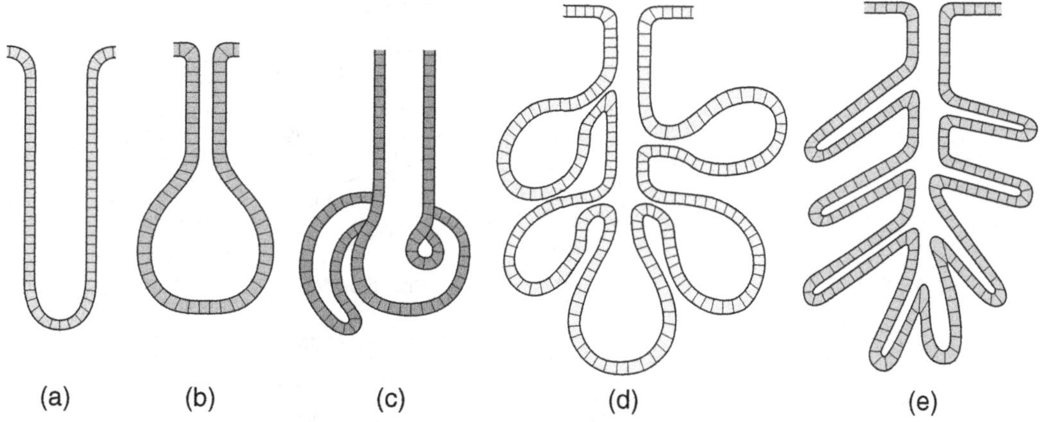

Figure 2.1 The different shapes of the exocrine gland. (a), (b) and (c) are simple glands. (a) Tubular glands found in the wall of the stomach and small intestine. (b) Saccular gland, e.g. the sebaceous glands in the skin. These are also called alveolar glands. (c) Coiled gland, e.g. the sweat glands in the nose and foot pads. (d) and (e) are compound glands. (d) Alveolar glands, e.g. salivary glands. (e) Tubular glands, e.g. duodenal glands.
(Reproduced with kind permission from CAW et al 2005).

Connective tissue

Key Points:

1. As the name suggests, connective tissue connects other body tissues together.
2. The types of connective tissue are diverse but they all have a framework, or matrix, in which all other components are situated.
3. There are five main types of connective tissue:
   a. Loose connective tissue; produced by fibroblasts, this white 'areolar' tissue is found subcutaneously as the *superficial fascia* and surrounding the organs.
   b. Dense connective tissue; produced by fibroblasts and infiltrated with collagen fibres to give it strength, this is found as scars, tendons, ligaments and surrounding muscles as the *deep fascia*.
   c. Cartilage; produced by chondroblasts, it is unlike the other connective tissues as it does not have a direct blood supply but a surrounding *perichondrium,* which provides the blood. Hyaline cartilage is the most frequently found but fibrocartilage is found in areas where great strength is needed, and elastic cartilage is found in areas requiring great elasticity.
   d. Blood (see Ch. 7, 'The Heart & Blood Vascular System, Lymphatic and Immune Systems', for more information).
   e. Bone (see Ch. 3, 'The Skeletal System', for more information).

Study

What is adipose tissue and where is it found? When would you find an excess of adipose tissue in an animal?

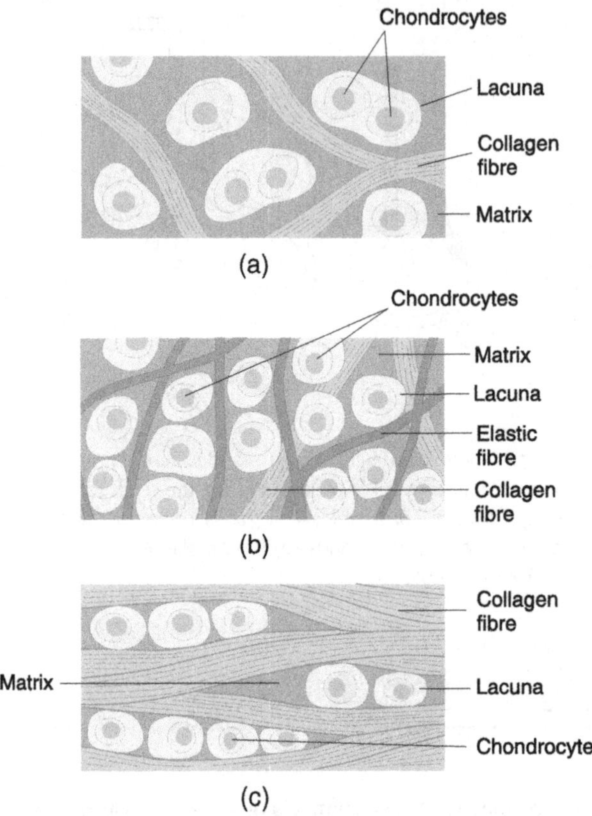

Figure 2.2 Structure of the different types of cartilage. (a) Hyaline cartilage. (b) Elastic cartilage. (c) Fibrocartilage. (Reproduced with kind permission from CAW et al 2005).

List the structures

Exercise 2.3 Place the following words into one of the three boxes in the chart below to categorize where each type of cartilage is found.

(1) Epiglottis
(2) Pinnae
(3) Costal cartilage
(4) Early fetal skeleton
(5) Intervertebral disc
(6) Joint sockets
(7) Articular surfaces of joints
(8) Rhinarium

Hyaline	Fibro	Elastic

Facts about body cavities

1. There are many cavities in the body, e.g. the oral and nasal cavities, but within the context of veterinary anatomy a body cavity is an area that is completely enclosed and lined with a serous membrane (see Body Tissues section in this chapter, for more information).
2. There are two major body cavities:
   a. the thoracic cavity
   b. the abdominal cavity.
3. The organs enclosed within body cavities are held in place by soft tissue ligaments attached to the body cavity wall.
4. The pericardium is also a body cavity, although this only contains one organ, the heart.

The thoracic cavity

Key Points:

1. The boundaries of the thoracic cavity are:
   a. laterally, the ribs and intercostal muscles
   b. cranially, the thoracic inlet, an oval opening parallel to the first rib pair
   c. caudally, the diaphragm
   d. dorsally, the hypaxial muscles and thoracic vertebrae
   e. ventrally, the sternum.
2. In cross-section, the thoracic cavity is oval, being wider dorsally than ventrally.
3. The serous lining of the thoracic cavity is the pleural membrane or pleura.
4. Pleura also lines the lungs and the mediastinum, creating two sacs known as the left and right pleural cavities.

List the structures

Exercise 2.4 List the structures contained within the thoracic cavity.

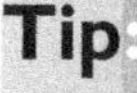

Don't confuse the pleural membrane and the pulmonary membrane!

The abdominal cavity

Key Points:

1. The abdominal cavity also includes the area sometimes called the pelvic cavity—there is no separation between them.
2. The boundaries of the abdominal cavity are:
   a. laterally, the abdominal oblique muscles and shaft of the ilium on either side
   b. cranially, the diaphragm
   c. caudally, the pelvic outlet which is closed off by the coccygeal and retractor ani muscles—the pelvic diaphragm

   d. dorsally, the hypaxial muscles and lumbar vertebrae
   e. ventrally, the abdominal oblique muscles, ischium and pubis on either side.
3. The abdominal cavity is separated into three major regions:
   a. the cranial abdominal region
   b. the middle abdominal region
   c. the caudal abdominal region.
4. The serous lining of the abdominal cavity is known as the peritoneal membrane or peritoneum.
5. The folds of the peritoneum dip down into the cavity to enclose and support the abdominal organs—these are called a mesentery, omentum or soft tissue ligament, depending on their structure:
   a. A mesentery is a wide peritoneal fold attaching organs to the abdominal wall and containing blood vessels, lymph vessels or nerves.
   b. An omentum is a wide peritoneal fold enclosing and attaching the stomach to other organs and the abdominal wall. The greater omentum – the largest omentum – contains a lot of fat.
   c. A soft tissue ligament runs from an organ to the abdominal wall or to another organ. It is narrow and contains few or no vessels.

List the structures

Exercise 2.5 List the structures contained within the abdominal cavity.

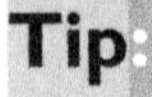

Don't confuse peritoneum and perineum!

Study

It is important to learn the position of the organs (viscera) in the body cavities. There are many ways to do this:

- take every opportunity to examine thoracic and abdominal radiographs
- assist with surgery
- assist with post-mortem examinations
- assist with manual palpations, e.g. bladder expression.

Activity

On the diagram below draw the boundaries of the thoracic and abdominal cavities. Next, sketch in the position of the major organs within each cavity. Why not enlarge by photocopying and stick it where you will regularly see it?

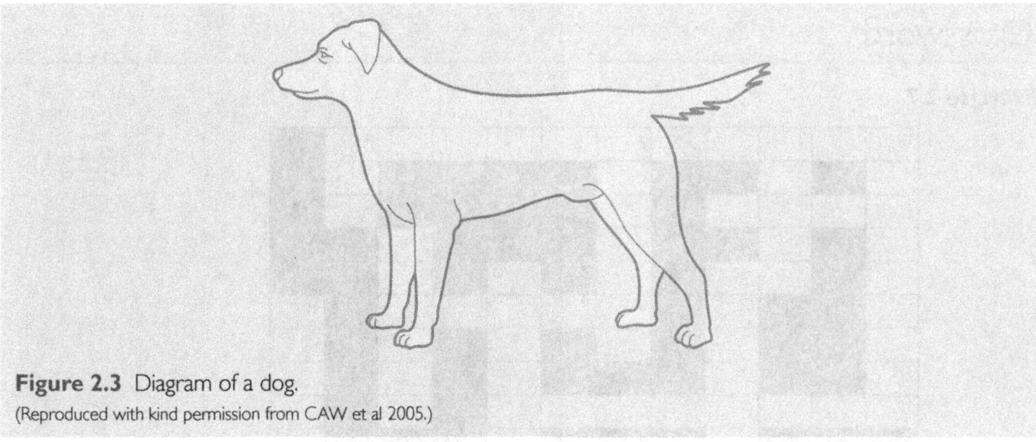

Figure 2.3 Diagram of a dog.
(Reproduced with kind permission from CAW et al 2005.)

General revision

Multiple choice questions – body tissues

Exercise 2.6

1. Mucous membrane is
   a. mucus-producing epithelial tissue
   b. mucus-producing cartilage
   c. serum-producing epithelial tissue
   d. serum-producing cartilage.
2. The pharynx is lined with
   a. simple squamous epithelial tissue
   b. cuboidal epithelial tissue
   c. transitional epithelial tissue
   d. stratified squamous epithelial tissue.
3. The pancreas is termed a mixed gland because
   a. it produces two secretions
   b. it has both endocrine and exocrine functions
   c. it joins ducts with another gland
   d. it is made of epithelial tissue and adipose tissue.
4. The prefix chondro- pertains to
   a. bone
   b. cartilage
   c. muscle
   d. hair.
5. Ligaments
   a. connect bone to epithelial tissue
   b. connect muscle to bone
   c. connect bone to bone
   d. connect epithelial tissue to muscle.

Tip: *Why not get together with fellow students and write some more questions for each other?*

Crossword

Exercise 2.7

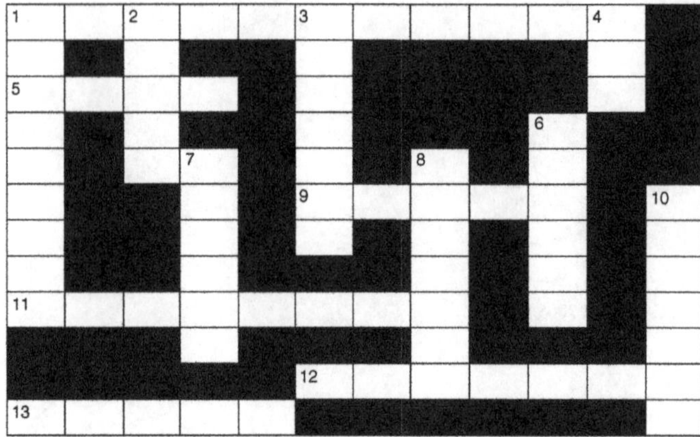

Across	**Down**
1. The lining of the heart, blood and lymph vessels.	1. This skeleton is hyaline cartilage.
5. The connective tissue with a rigid matrix.	2. This connective tissue forms ligaments.
9. The body tissue that transmits impulses.	3. The secretion from an endocrine gland.
11. Another name for cubical epithelial tissue.	4. Prefix pertaining to muscle.
12. The protein that infiltrates skin.	6. This is lined with transitional epithelial tissue.
13. Dense connective tissue structures that form over wounds.	7. The structure that connects muscle to bone.
	8. Another term for loose connective tissue.
	10. The most commonly found cartilage.

Activity

Design a poster on A3 paper depicting the different types of body tissues. Use large labels and bold colours. When it is complete, stick it where you will regularly read it. Why not on a kitchen cupboard?

Multiple choice questions – body cavities

Exercise 2.8

1. Serous fluid is:
   a. a red-coloured watery fluid
   b. a straw-coloured watery fluid
   c. a red-coloured mucoid fluid
   d. a straw-coloured mucoid fluid.
2. The diaphragm separates the:
   a. exterior and the thoracic cavity
   b. thoracic and abdominal cavities
   c. thoracic and pelvic cavities
   d. exterior and the abdominal cavity.

3. The major abdominal organ that is not enclosed within the peritoneum is the:
   a. liver
   b. spleen
   c. stomach
   d. kidney.
4. Which of the following structures is the most cranial in the abdominal cavity?
   a. stomach
   b. liver
   c. urinary bladder
   d. duodenum.
5. Which of the following structures lies alongside the duodenum and stomach?
   a. pancreas
   b. spleen
   c. kidney
   d. ovary.
6. Which of the following structures lies between the lobes of the liver?
   a. pancreas
   b. ovary
   c. kidney
   d. gall bladder.
7. Which part of the digestive tract runs through the diaphragm?
   a. pharynx
   b. oesophagus
   c. stomach
   d. ileum.
8. When empty, the urinary bladder is positioned within the:
   a. thoracic cavity
   b. cranial abdominal region
   c. middle abdominal region
   d. caudal abdominal region.

Tip: *Why not get together with fellow students and write some more questions for each other?*

CHAPTER 3

The skeletal system

LEARNING **Objectives**

This chapter will help you to revise the following:

- facts and functions of the skeletal system
- bone tissue and formation
- endochondral ossification in the long bones
- bone types and structure
- the skeleton in general
- the skull
- the vertebrae
- the ribs and sternum
- the pelvis
- the long bones of the limbs
- the manus and the pes
- joints
- anatomical landmarks related to the skeleton.

There is a general revision section at the end of the chapter.

Facts and functions of the skeletal system

1. The skeletal system provides rigidity and support for the body.
2. It is a site for muscle attachment to allow leverage during movement.
3. Some of the bones have a protective function.
4. It is a site of mineral storage, e.g. calcium.
5. The myeloid tissue, or bone marrow, is responsible for the production of all blood cells, although some cells develop and mature in other body systems. (See Ch. 7, 'The Heart and Blood Vascular System, and Lymphatic and Immune Systems', for information about lymphocytes).
6. The prefix denoting bone is *ost–*.

Bone tissue and formation

Key Points:

1. Bone tissue is made up of:
   a. 25% water
   b. 45% organic matter
   c. 30% mineral (mainly Ca and P).
2. There are four main types of bone cell:
   a. osteoprogenitor cells—precursors of osteoblasts, which line the inner surface of periosteum
   b. osteoblasts—the bone-forming cells that make up the bone matrix and become osteocytes once they have matured
   c. osteocytes—the mature bone cells that maintain the bone matrix
   d. osteoclasts—the bone-resorbing cells that form the medullary cavity of long bones.
3. Mature bone tissue is made up of osteocytes lying in concentric circles and surrounded by a calcified matrix—an haversian system.
4. Compact bone has haversian systems that run parallel to each other and are closely packed together.
5. Cancellous (spongy) bone has haversian systems that are not parallel or uniform in appearance.

6. There are three different types of bone formation (ossification):
    a. heteroplastic—bone formed in tissue other than the skeleton, i.e. the os penis, the U-shaped bone found in the penis of most animals
    b. intramembranous—bone formed inside ('intra') a membrane ('membranous'), e.g. the flat bones of the skull
    c. endochondral—bone formed when the innermost ('endo') cartilage ('chondral') cells move outwards and become calcified, e.g. the long bones of the limbs.

Activity

Exercise 3.1 Below is a diagram of an haversian system. From the selection, add the correct labels to the diagram.

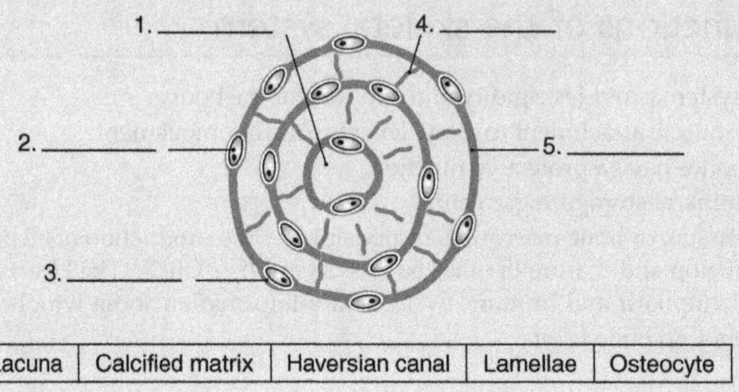

Lacuna	Calcified matrix	Haversian canal	Lamellae	Osteocyte

Figure 3.1 An haversian system.

Endochondral ossification in the long bones

Key Points:

1. Mostly complete prior to birth.
2. Continues after birth from cartilage plates (growth plates) found between the diaphysis and epiphyses of the long bone.
3. Completes when the animal reaches full size, so this will vary between breeds.
4. The proximal epiphyseal plate is the first to begin ossification and the last to fuse.

Activity

Exercise 3.2 Below is a diagram of the process of endochondral ossification. From the selection, add the correct label to each stage in the ossification process.

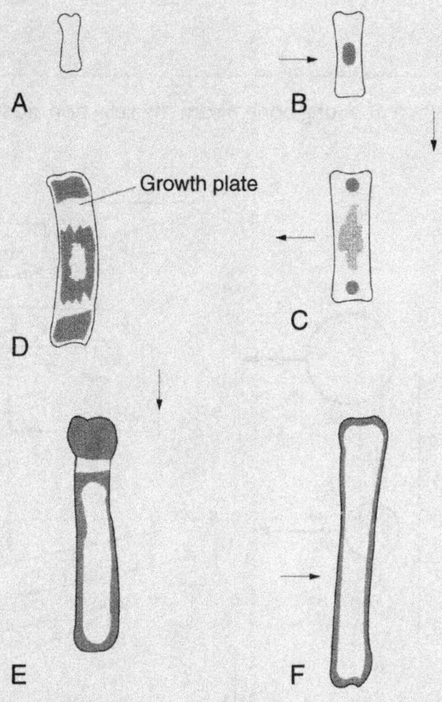

First growth plate fuses. Medullary cavity continues into epiphysis. Growth is only now possible at proximal growth plate	Cartilage model in fetus	Ossification begins from primary centre of ossification in shaft (diaphysis)
Proximal growth plate fuses. Bone growth ceases	Ossification continues in diaphysis and epiphyses. Osteoclasts begin to break down bone in shaft to form marrow cavity	Ossification in shaft continues. Secondary centres of ossification appear in epiphyses

Figure 3.2 Endochondral ossification.
(Reproduced with kind permission from Lane & Cooper 1999.)

Bone types and structure

Key Points:

1. Most bones have an outer membrane (periosteum), an outer layer of compact bone and an inner layer of cancellous (spongy) bone.
2. Bones are classified according to their shape:
   a. flat bones, e.g. most of the skull bones
   b. short bones, e.g. carpal bones

c. irregular bones, e.g. vertebrae
d. sesamoid bones—bones found in tendons or ligaments, such as the patella
e. long bones, e.g. femur or humerus. These bones have a medullary cavity filled with bone marrow and hyaline cartilage at their epiphyses.

Activity

Exercise 3.3 Below is a diagram of a long bone. From the selection, add the correct labels to the diagram.

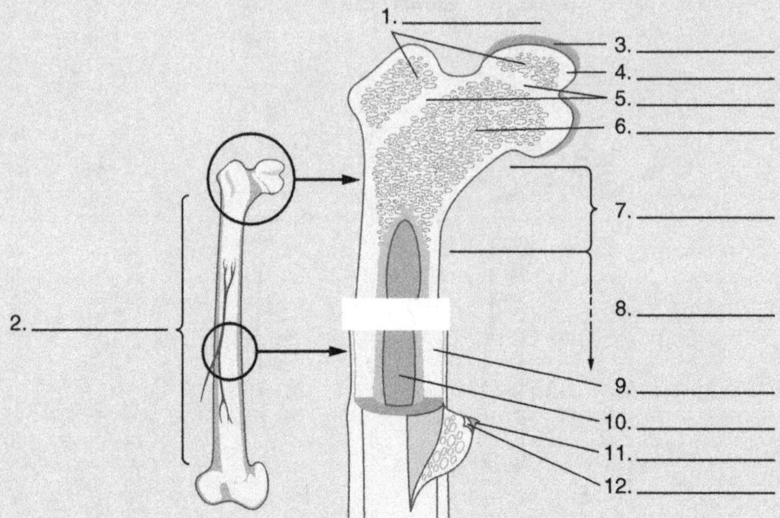

Cancellous bone trabeculae	Marrow cavity (medullary cavity)	Hyaline articular cartilage	Periosteum osteogenic layer	Epiphyseal lines	Compact bone
Epiphysis	Compact bone	Metaphysis	Diaphysis	Diaphysis (shaft)	Fibrous layer

Figure 3.3 The structure of a long bone.
(Reproduced with kind permission from CAW et al 2005.)

Link the words

Exercise 3.4 Match the description of the features of bones in the left-hand column to the correct definition in the right-hand column, by drawing a line to link them.

(1)Another name for the joints of the flat bones	(2)Process
(3)A small depression in the bone; often contains structures within it or is an area for muscle attachment	(4)Foramen

(Continued)

(5)A small nodule or rounded prominence on a bone	(6)Sulcus
(7)A rounded prominence found at the end of a bone, which articulates with another bone	(8)Notch
(9)A cleft or groove	(10)Fossa
(11)A bony projection	(12)Condyle
(13)A dip or dent in the bone, often an area for articulation with another bone	(14)Sinus
(15)A hole in the bone through which blood vessels or nerves pass	(16)Tubercle
(17)A long narrow ridge of bone	(18)Suture
(19)An air filled cavity within a bone	(20)Crest

The skeleton in general

Key Points:

1. The skeleton's functions are to protect, support and aid movement.
2. Bone marrow is found in the spaces between cancellous bone and in the medullary cavity of long bones. It is important for blood cell production.
3. The *axial* skeleton comprises the skull, mandible, hyoid bone, vertebrae, ribs and sternebrae.
4. The *appendicular* skeleton comprises the bones of the forelimb (known as the thoracic limb) and the hindlimb (known as the pelvic limb).
5. The *splanchnic* skeleton comprises the os penis.

Mnemonic

To remember the components of the axial skeleton

Very **s**mall **m**urderers **h**ave **r**eally **s**mall **ax**es!

V: Vertebrae
S: Skull
M: Mandible
H: Hyoid bone
R: Ribs
S: Sternum
Ax: To remind you this is the axial skeleton!

Activity

Exercise 3.5 Below is a diagram of a skeleton. From the selection, add the correct labels to the diagram.

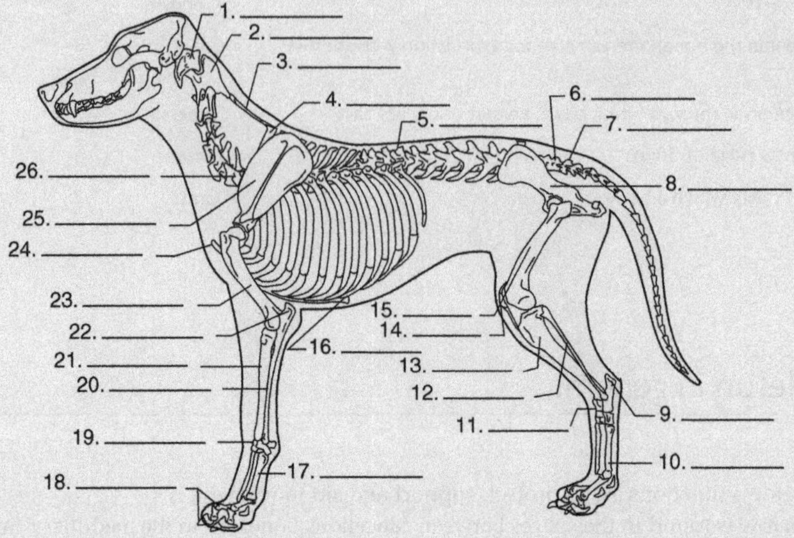

Patella	Ligamentum nuchae	Radius	Sacrum
Metatarsal bones	Scapula	Metacarpal bones	Femur
Humerus	Tarsal bones	L1 first lumbar vertebra	Ulna
C7 last cervical vertebra	Cy1 first vertebra (coccygeal)	Carpal bones	C2, axis
Calcaneus (point of hock)	Os coxae (pelvis)	T1 first thoracic vertebra	Tibia
Cranial end of sternum (manubrium)	Proximal, middle, and distal phalanges	Caudal end (xiphoid) of sternum	C1, atlas
Fibula	Olecranon (point of elbow)		

Figure 3.4 The canine skeleton.
(Reproduced with kind permission from Colville & Bassert 2002.)

The skull

Key Points:

1. The skull consists mainly of flat bones.
2. It is split into two main areas—the cranium and the jaws.
3. The primary job of the cranium is to protect the brain, eyes and ears.
4. The jaws provide areas for muscle attachment and anchorage for teeth.
5. The paranasal sinuses are found in the maxillary and frontal bones.

6. The foramen magnum allows the spinal cord to enter the cranium.
7. The three main skull shapes in dogs are:
   a. brachycephalic—found in short-nosed breeds such as the bulldog
   b. mesaticephalic—found in medium-shaped breeds such as the beagle
   c. dolichocephalic—found in very long-nosed breeds such as the borzoi.

Activity

Below is a diagram of a skull. To make a jigsaw puzzle, follow the steps below:

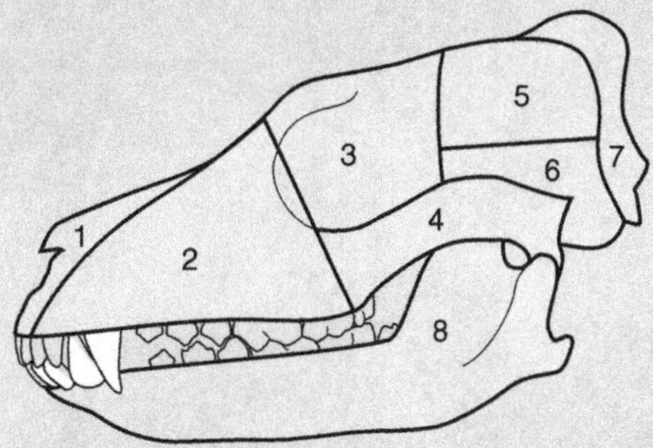

1. Incisive or premaxilla 2. Maxilla 3. Frontal 4. Zygomatic arch
5. Parietal 6. Temporal 7. Occipital region 8. Mandible

Figure 3.5 Jigsaw puzzle of an animal's skull.
(Adapted, with kind permission, from CAW et al 2005.)

1. Photocopy the diagram.
2. Colour in and label the photocopy.
3. Cut out each individual bone.
4. Keep the pieces safe! You can use the puzzle several times to help you learn skull anatomy.

Activity

There are some differences between the skull of the dog and the skull of the cat. Write them below:

The vertebrae

Key Points:

1. There are five different types of vertebra.
2. All vertebrae share common features but their shape changes according to their position in the body and the function they must perform.

3. Due to their position in the body, the atlas (C1) and axis (C2) are highly specialized. They must be able to withstand and support a significant amount of pressure and weight whilst still allowing a high degree of movement.
4. Vertebrae are separated by intervertebral discs that are made from fibrocartilage on the outside (anulus fibrosus) with a gel-like centre (nucleus pulposus). These discs allow increased movement and also act as protective 'shock absorbers' for the vertebral column.
5. The spinal cord runs down the centre of the vertebrae, in the vertebral foramen. It gradually tapers just cranial to the sacral vertebrae.

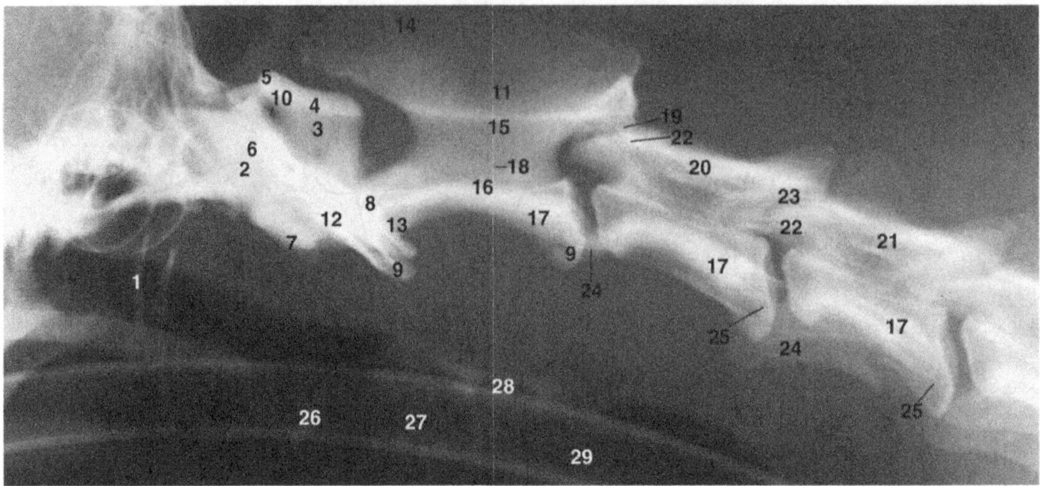

Figure 3.6 Lateral radiograph of the cranial cervical portion of the canine spine. (1) Stylohyoid bone. (2) Occipital condyle. (3) First cervical vertebra (atlas). (4) Dorsal arch. (5) Dorsal tubercle. (6) Border of cranial articular surface. (7) Ventral arch. (8) Border of caudal articular surface. (9) Transverse process. (10) Lateral vertebral foramen. (11) Second cervical vertebra (axis). (12) Dens. (13) Cranial articular surface. (14) Spinous process. (15) Dorsal border of vertebral foramen/canal. (16) Ventral border of vertebral foramen/canal. (17) Body. (18) Transverse foramen. (19) Articular processes. (20) Third cervical vertebra. (21) Fourth cervical vertebra. (22) Cranial articular process. (23) Caudal articular process. (24) Cranial extension of transverse process. (25) Caudal extension of transverse process. (26) Thyrohyoid bone. (27) Thyroid cartilage. (28) Cricoid cartilage. (29) Trachea (with endotracheal tube).

(Reproduced with kind permission from Boyd 2001.)

Look it up

Exercise 3.6 Complete the chart below by writing the correct numbers of each type of vertebra in the boxes.

Cervical	Thoracic	Lumbar	Sacral	Coccygeal
(1)	(2)	(3)	(4) (fused)	(5)

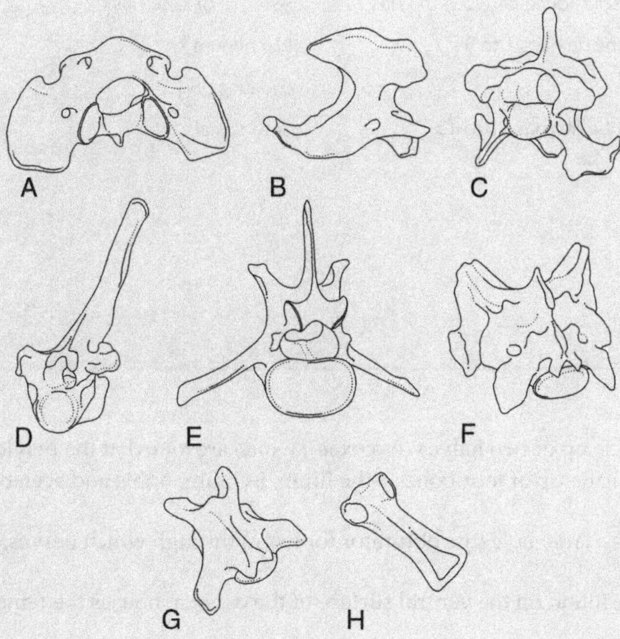

Figure 3.7 The differences between vertebrae. (a) Atlas; (b) axis; (c) cervical vertebra; (d) thoracic vertebra; (e) lumbar vertebra; (f) sacral vertebrae (fused); (g) proximal coccygeal vertebra; (h) distal coccygeal vertebra. (Adapted with kind permission from Evans 1993.)

The ribs and sternum

Key Points:

1. The ribs and sternum serve to protect the thoracic cavity and aid respiration.
2. There are 13 pairs of ribs; proximally, one pair attaches to the costal foveae of each thoracic vertebra.
3. Each rib has a proximal bony part and a distal cartilaginous part. They meet at the costochondral junction.
4. Distally, rib pair numbers 1 to 9 attach to the sternum.
5. Rib number 9 is the longest rib.
6. Distally, rib pairs 10 to 12 attach to the next cranial rib.
7. Rib number 13 is not attached distally.
8. There are eight sternebrae.

Link the words

Exercise 3.7 To test your knowledge of the terminology of the ribs and sternum, match the description in the left-hand column to the correct definition in the right-hand column, by drawing a line to link them.

(1)Sternebra number 1	(2)Sternal or true ribs
(3)Term used to describe rib pair 13	(4)Xiphoid process or xiphisternum

(Continued)

(5)The name of the muscles found between the ribs	(6)Asternal or false ribs
(7)Terms used to describe rib pairs 1 to 9	(8)Manubrium
(9)Sternebra number 8	(10)Floating rib
(11)Terms used to describe rib pairs 10 to 13	(12)Intercostal

The pelvis

Key Points:

1. The pelvis is made up of two halves (os coxae), which are joined at the pelvic symphysis.
2. Each os coxa is made up of four bones—the ilium, ischium, pubis and acetabular bone, which are fused together.
3. Each os coxa has a large hole (the obturator foramen) through which nerves, blood vessels and muscles pass.
4. The acetabulum, found on the ventral surface of the os coxa, houses the femoral head to form the hip joint.

Activity

Exercise 3.8 Below is a diagram of the pelvis of a dog. From the selection, add the correct labels to the diagram.

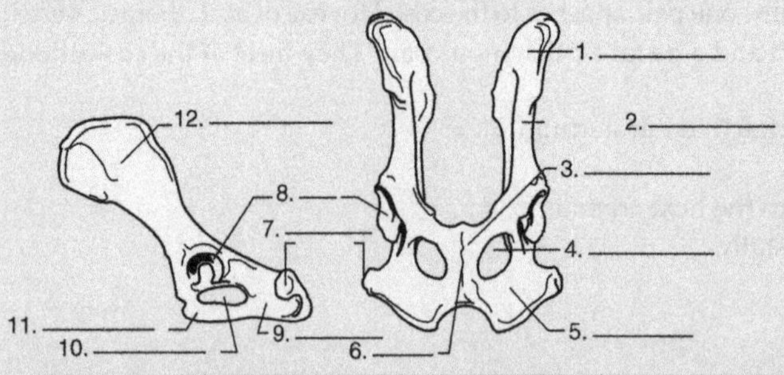

Obturator foramen	Wing of ilium	Ischial tuberosity	Ilium	Ischium	Pubic symphysis
Acetabulum	Pubis	Ischium	Pubis	Obturator foramen	Wing of ilium

Figure 3.8 The canine pelvis.
(Reproduced with kind permission from Colville & Bassert 2002.)

The long bones of the limbs

Key Points:

1. The medullary cavity and the spaces in cancellous bone contain bone marrow, which is important for blood cell production.
2. The long bones of the limbs are the last bones in the body to complete ossification.

What am I?

Exercise 3.9 Name the bones described below, writing the correct answer in the space provided.

A bone of the thoracic limb, my proximal end forms part of the elbow joint. Distally, my end is concave and has the styloid process extending into the carpal area. (1)

I am a very large straight bone. Proximally, the greater trochanter lies laterally. Distally, the lateral and medial condyles form part of the stifle joint. (2)

My proximal end is triangular in cross-section and a crest of bone projects cranially. Distally, I articulate with the tarsus. (3)

I am a large bone with a twist in my diaphysis. Distally, a large supracondylarforamen can be found into which slots the anconeal process of the ulna. (4)

I am a very thin bone, which lies caudal to the tibia at my proximal end and lateral to the tibia at my distal end. (5)

The longest bone in the body, I lie on the caudal aspect of the limb proximally and on the lateral aspect distally. The surface, which forms part of the elbow joint, has a distinctive shape due to the half-moon-shaped trochlear notch. (6)

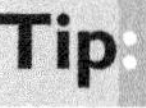

Write some more descriptions and test fellow students!

The manus and the pes

Key Points:

1. The manus comprises the carpus, metacarpus and digits.
2. The pes comprises the tarsus, metatarsus and digits.
3. Digits are always counted and numbered medially to laterally, so digit number 1 is the 'dew-claw' and is always counted, even if it is absent.

Activity

Exercise 3.10 Below is a diagram of the manus. From the selection, add the correct labels to the diagram.

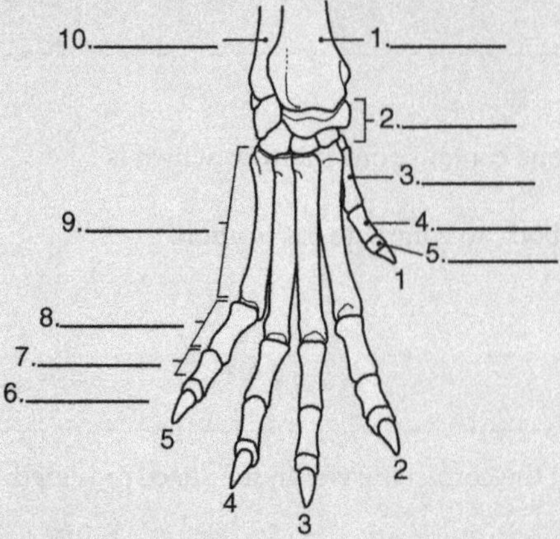

Proximal phalanges	Medial phalanx of digit 1	Medial phalanges	Radius	Distal phalanges
Proximal phalanx of digit 1 (sometimes labelled metacarpal 1)	4 Metacarpal bones (numbered 2–5)	Distal phalanx of digit 1 with the ungual process that forms the nail core	Ulna	2 Rows of carpal bones

Figure 3.9 The manus.
(Adapted with kind permission from Hine 1988.)

Activity

Exercise 3.11 Below is a diagram of the pes. From the selection, add the correct labels to the diagram.

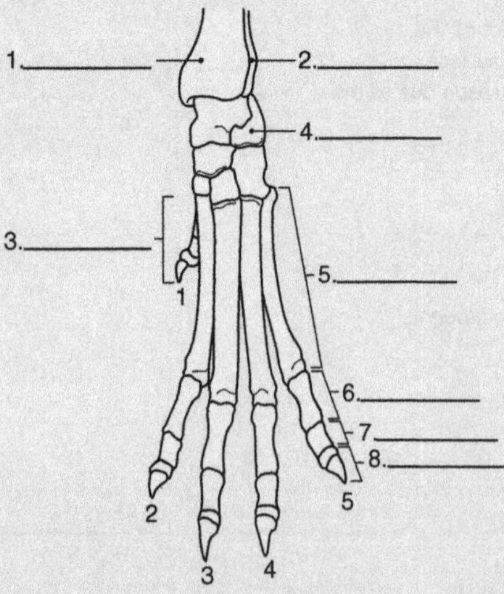

Distal phalanges (with ungual process)	Proximal phalanges	Fibular tarsal of calcaneus which makes point of hock	Fibula
Phalanges of dew claw attached to tarsus	Tibia	Medial phalanges	Metatarsals

Figure 3.10 The pes.
(Adapted with kind permission from Hine 1988.)

Joints

Key Points:

1. A joint is the area where two or more bones meet.
2. The prefix denoting a joint is *arth–*.
3. Joints are classified according to their structure. Sometimes they are described in terms of the type of movement they produce (e.g. hinge or gliding).

Activity

Exercise 3.12 Below is a diagram of a synovial joint. From the selection, add the correct labels to the diagram.

Bone

1. ______
2. ______
3. ______
4. ______
5. ______

Bone

Fibrous membrane (outer)	Periosteum	Articular cartilage
Synovial fluid	Synovial membrane (inner)	

Figure 3.11 The synovial joint.
(Reproduced with kind permission from Bowden & Masters 2001.)

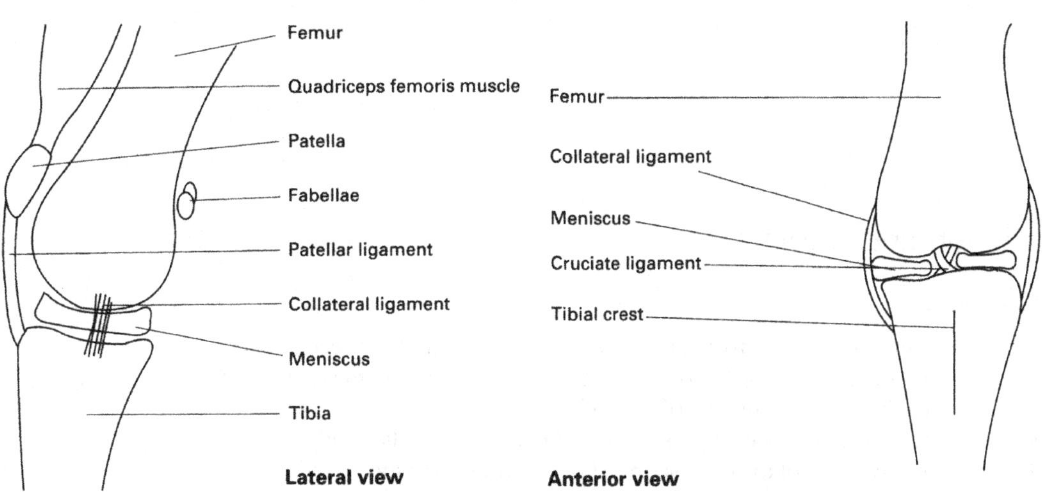

Figure 3.12 The stifle joint.
(Reproduced with kind permission from Lane & Cooper 1999.)

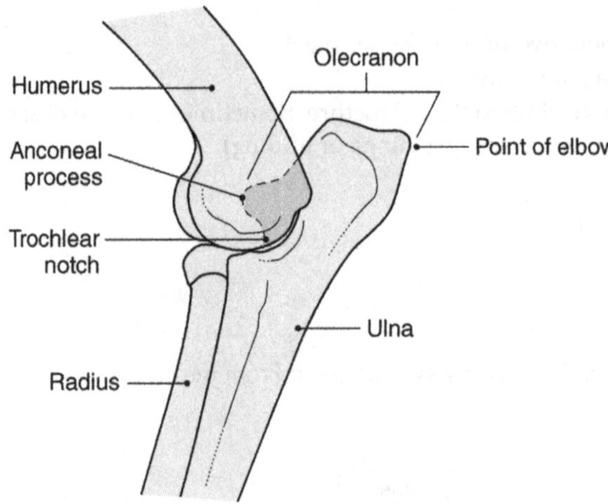

Figure 3.13 The elbow joint.

What am I?

Exercise 3.13 Categorize the joints below, writing the correct answer in the space provided.

Sutures of the skull	(1)
Temporomandibular junction	(2)
Atlanto-occipital joint	(3)
Junction of L2 and L3	(4)
Junction of T5 and T6	(5)
Elbow	(6)
Hip	(7)
Pelvic symphysis	(8)
Stifle	(9)

Movement of joints

Key Points:

1. Flexion and extension—decreasing and increasing the angle between bones.
2. Abduction and adduction—moving the body part away from the midline of the body and moving it towards the midline of the body
3. Circumduction—movement of one end of a bone in a circular motion.
4. Rotation—twisting of the bone so that it faces a different aspect.

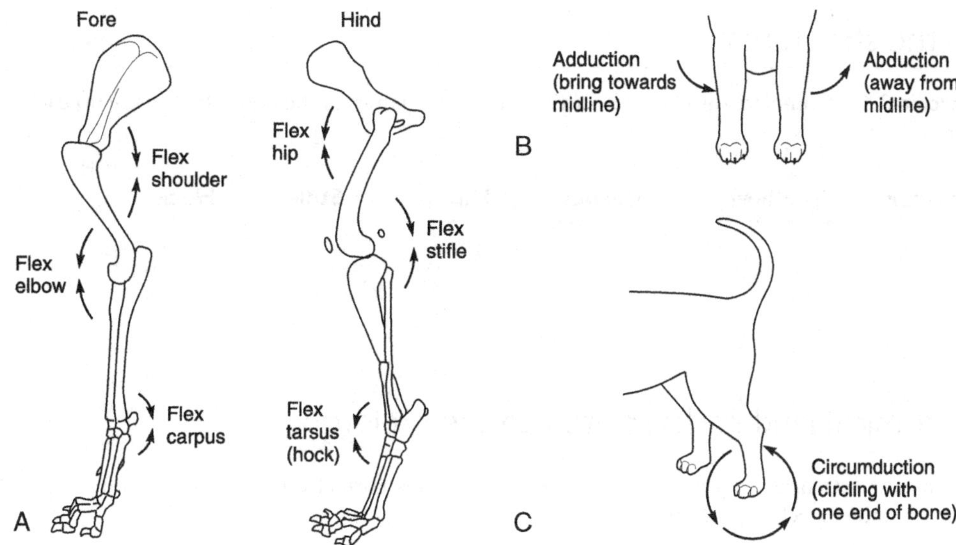

Figure 3.14 Joint movements.
(Reproduced with kind permission from Bowden & Masters 2001.)

Tip: *On an obliging animal, practise these movements. This will help you to understand how different joints move!*

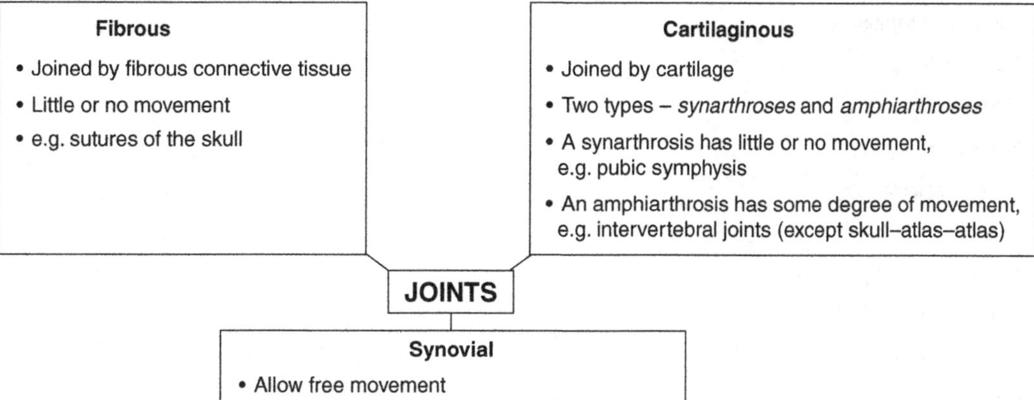

Figure 3.15 Classification of joints by their structures.

List the structures

Exercise 3.14 Complete the chart by writing down the names of the bones that make up each joint.

Shoulder	Elbow	Carpus	Hip	Stifle	Hock
(1)	(2)	(3)	(4)	(5)	(6)

Anatomical landmarks related to the skeleton

Anatomical landmarks are often used to position animals correctly for radiographs or to perform diagnostic and corrective procedures.

Activity

On an obliging animal, find the following anatomical landmarks.

Landmark	Notes
Saggital crest	
Atlanto-occipital junction	
Thoracolumbar junction	
Costal arch	
Xiphisternum	
Manubrium	
Spine of scapula	
Olecranon	
Accessory carpal	
Wing of ilium	
Ischial tuberosity	
Calcaneus	

Tip: *Spend some time looking at radiographs of the skeleton. Test yourself to see if you can name all the bones and joints on the X-rays.*

General revision

Multiple choice questions

Exercise 3.15

1. Bone resorbing cells that form the medullary cavity are called:
   a. osteoprogenitor cells
   b. osteoblasts
   c. osteocytes
   d. osteoclasts.
2. The flat bones of the skull develop by:
   a. heteroplastic ossification
   b. intramembranous ossification
   c. endochondral ossification
   d. pathologic ossification.
3. The globe of the eye is contained within the:
   a. orbit
   b. turbinate bones
   c. incisive bone
   d. occipit.
4. The axis is vertebra number:
   a. C1
   b. T1
   c. C2
   d. T2.
5. The vertebrae with the tallest dorsal (spinous) processes are the:
   a. cervical
   b. thoracic
   c. lumbar
   d. coccygeal.
6. The rib pair attaching to the manubrium is number:
   a. 1
   b. 5
   c. 9
   d. 13.
7. The ungual process is found on:
   a. the accessory carpal
   b. metacarpal one
   c. metatarsal two
   d. the distal phalanx.
8. The acromion process is found on the:
   a. mandible
   b. pelvis
   c. femur
   d. scapula.

9. The large hole in the os coxa is the:
   a. obturator foramen
   b. vertebral foramen
   c. foramen magnum
   d. foramen ovale.
10. The anticlinal vertebra is
    a. C3
    b. T7
    c. T11
    d. S3.

Tip: *Why not get together with fellow students and write some more questions for each other?*

Activity

Exercise 3.16 True or false? If the statement is false, write the corrected statement in the relevant space.

Statement	True or false
The forelimb has no bony attachment to the body	(1)
The mandibular symphysis is a synovial joint	(2)
The clavicle is rarely found in the dog	(3)
There are nine sternebrae	(4)
The radiocarpal joint rotates to a greater degree in the cat than the dog	(5)
The tibial tarsal bone is also known as the talus	(6)
The os penis is part of the appendicular skeleton	(7)
The tympanic bullae are found on the ventral aspect of the skull	(8)

Skeletal crossword

Exercise 3.17

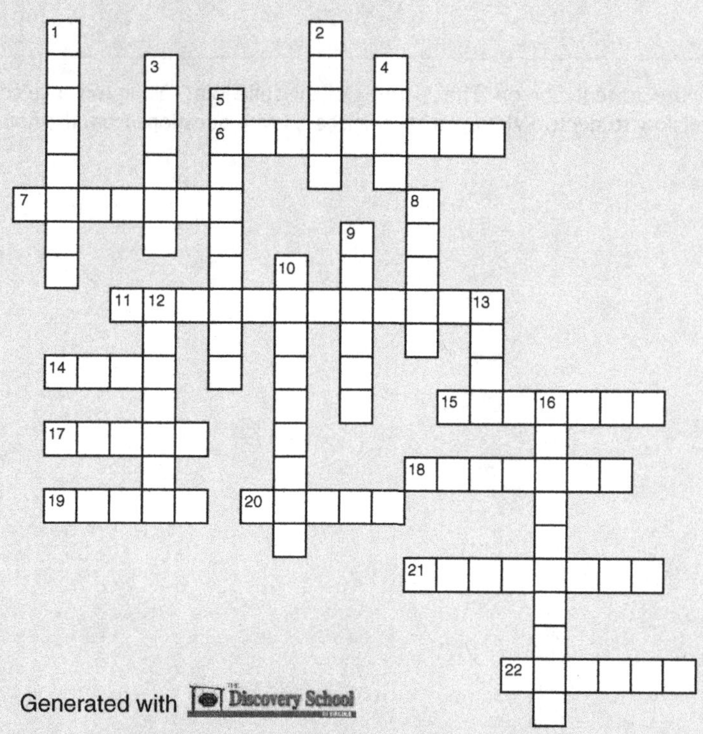

Across

6. Moving a part away from the midline.
7. The name for the ribs and sternum.
11. The process of bone formation.
14. The longest bone in the dog.
15. Digit number one.
17. This bone's head sits in the acetabulum.
18. True ribs.
19. The colour of synovial fluid.
20. Number of sternebrae.
21. Joint between the scapula and humerus.
22. The abdominal vertebrae.

Down

1. Another name for the premaxilla.
2. One of the bones of the pelvis.
3. Relating to the ribs.
4. The prefix denoting a joint.
5. These systems make up bone tissue.
8. An organ protected by the cranium.
9. Term meaning passageway or opening.
10. The bone shaft.
12. The most proximal bone of the forelimb.
13. The number of sternal ribs.
16. Another term for spongy bone.

Tip: *Have you seen a word or term you don't understand? Don't ignore it, look it up!*

Activity

Prepare a five-minute presentation on 'The anatomy of the stifle joint'. Your audience could be friends, family or fellow students. When you have finished, invite questions from the floor!

CHAPTER 4

The muscular system

LEARNING Objectives

This chapter will help you to revise the following:

- facts and functions of muscle tissue
- contraction of skeletal muscle
- the skeletal muscles
- the diaphragm
- tendons.

There is a general revision section at the end of the chapter.

Facts and functions of muscle tissue

1. The prefix denoting muscle tissue is *myo–*.
2. There are three types of muscle tissue:
   a. Cardiac muscle—highly specialized tissue that makes up the heart wall (myocardium) and pumps blood around the body. It is stimulated by pacemaker cells within the myocardium. Contractions are controlled by the autonomic nervous system (ANS).
   b. Involuntary muscle—also called unstriated or smooth muscle. Found in the viscera (internal organs) and blood vessel walls, its contractions are controlled by the ANS. Often, it contracts in a rhythmic wave-like motion to move substances along a tract (peristalsis), e.g. in the wall of the small intestine.
   c. Voluntary muscle—also called striated or skeletal muscle. This makes up the bulk of the body's musculature and it is the only type of muscle that the animal can consciously control (hence voluntary). It plays a major part in skeletal support, locomotion, production of body heat and control of body temperature by 'shivering'.

List the structures

Exercise 4.1 Place the following words under one of the three headings below to categorize the type of muscle found in each area.

(1)Bladder wall	(2)Stomach wall	(3)Jugular vein
(4)Stifle flexor	(5)Cephalic vein	(6)Carpal flexor
(7)Myocardium	(8)Small intestine	(9)Muscles of facial expression

Cardiac	Involuntary	Voluntary

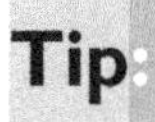

It's usually easy to work out what type of muscle tissue would be found in a certain area. Just ask yourself 'Can the animal consciously move the part?' If the answer is yes, then it must be voluntary muscle!

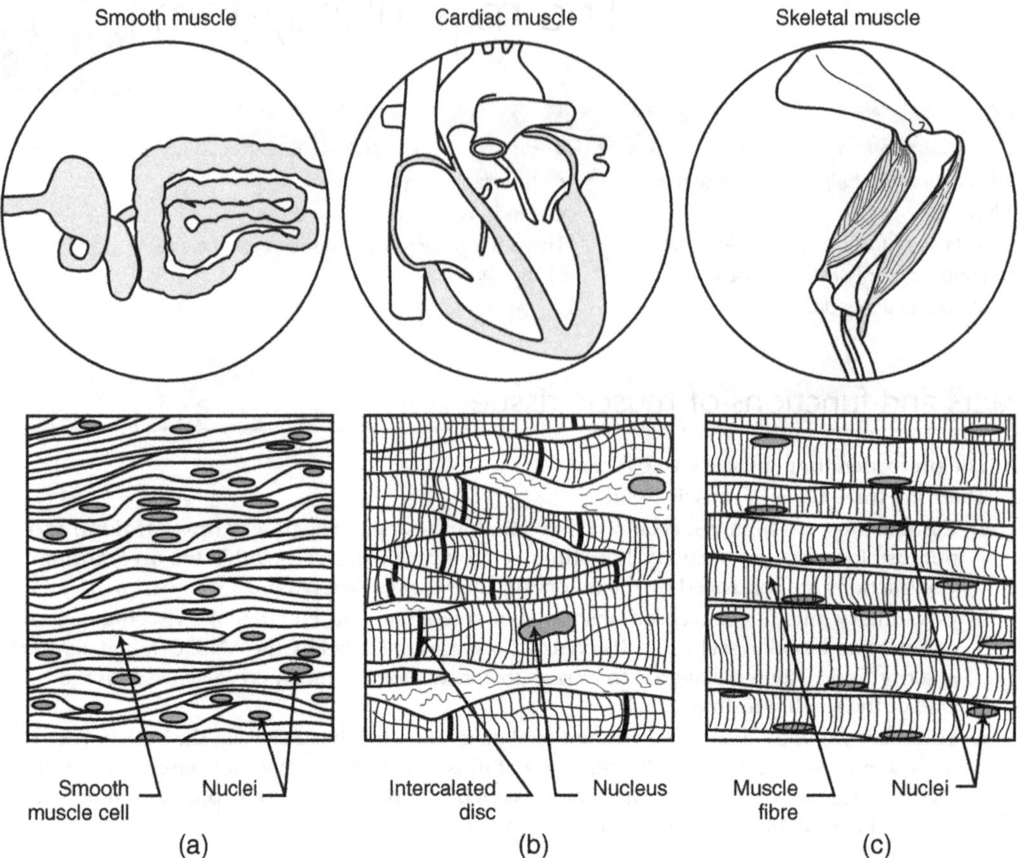

Figure 4.1 Diagrams of different muscle tissues. (a) Involuntary or smooth muscle. (b) Cardiac muscle. (c) Voluntary or skeletal muscle.

(Reproduced with kind permission from Colville & Bassert 2002.)

Contraction of voluntary (skeletal) muscle

Key Points:

1. Skeletal muscles are activated by nerve impulses—one nerve fibre innervates several muscle fibres (motor unit).
2. The size of a motor unit depends on the intricacy of movement needed—intrinsic muscles carrying out finer movements have a smaller number of muscle fibres to each nerve fibre than the extrinsic muscles, which have larger motor units.
3. A motor unit either contracts or doesn't contract (i.e. it cannot contract a little way). The strength of contraction in the muscle as a whole is determined by the number of motor units stimulated.

Link the words

Exercise 4.2 Match the description in the left-hand column to the correct definition in the right-hand column by drawing a line to link them.

(1)One nerve fibre innervating several muscle fibres	(2)Epaxial
(3)A type of contraction where the length of the muscle changes but not the tone	(4)Motor unit
(5)A muscle restricted to one body part, which changes the shape of that part	(6)Sarcolemma
(7)Term for the muscles found beneath the vertebral column	(8)Sarcomere
(9)A type of contraction where the tone of the muscle changes but not the length	(10)Intrinsic
(11)An individual contractile unit of which skeletal muscle is composed	(12)Extrinsic
(13)Term for the muscles found above the vertebral column	(14)Isometric
(15)A muscle that spans more than one body part and changes the position of that part in relation to the rest of the body	(16)Hypaxial
(17)The cell membrane that encloses muscle cells	(18)Isotonic

How a muscle contracts

1. Each sarcomere is made up of a dark band (myosin) and light bands (actin).
2. There is a natural attraction between myosin and actin which, during relaxation, is prevented by a certain chemical environment.
3. The contraction process starts when a nerve impulse arrives at the neuromuscular junction. A chain of events occurs which causes the release of calcium ions.
4. The calcium ions change the chemical environment to allow the natural attraction between myosin and actin to occur. This causes the sarcomere to shorten—contraction.
5. For separation of the myosin and actin to occur, energy is required in the form of adenosine triphosphate (ATP).
6. It is the depletion of ATP after death that prevents the separation of myosin and actin, thus causing rigor mortis.

The skeletal muscles

Key Points:

1. The muscles of the skeleton are all voluntary (striated).
2. All muscles have a basic structure:
   a. Tendon of origin, which is always the more proximal or medial tendon and does not move greatly during contraction. There are usually only one or two tendons of origin.

b. The main belly of the muscle tissue. There may be more than one belly.
c. The tendon of insertion, which is always the more distal or lateral tendon and tends to move considerably during contraction. There may be more than one tendon of insertion.

3. Skeletal muscles always attach to one or more bones at both ends.

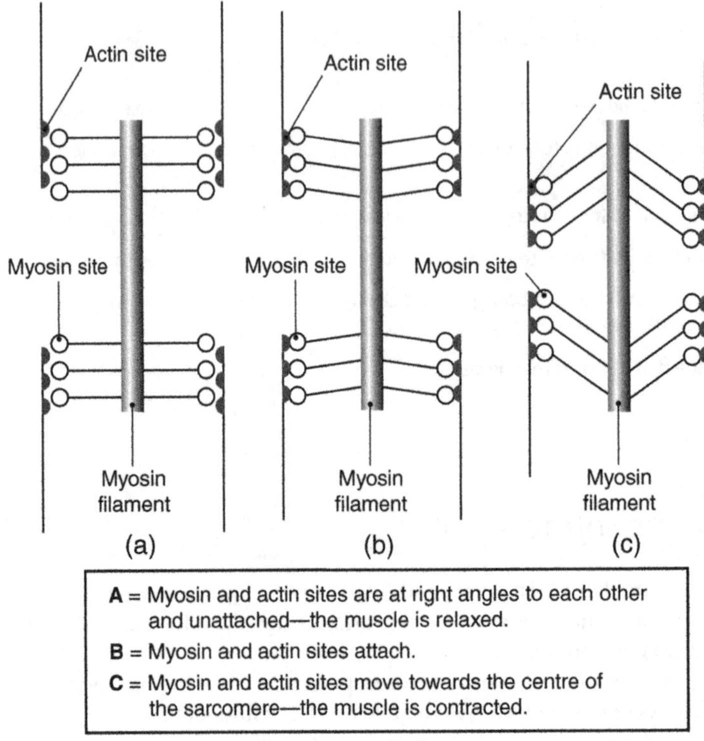

Figure 4.2 Diagram of sarcomere relaxed and contracted.

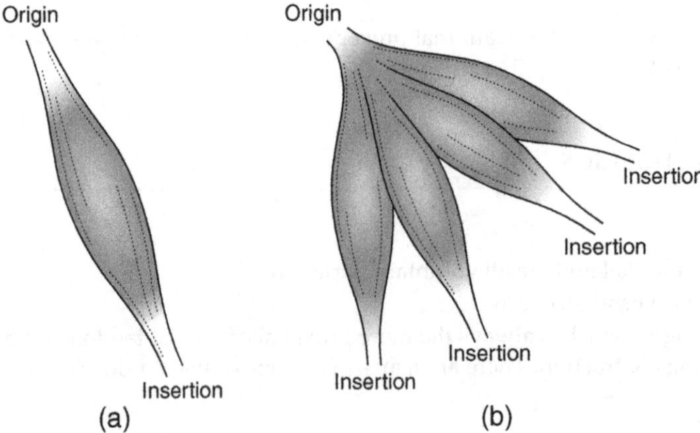

Figure 4.3 Diagram of (a) simple and (b) compound skeletal muscles.

Below is a diagram of the muscles of the head. Note that the digistracus is on the medial aspect of the mandible.

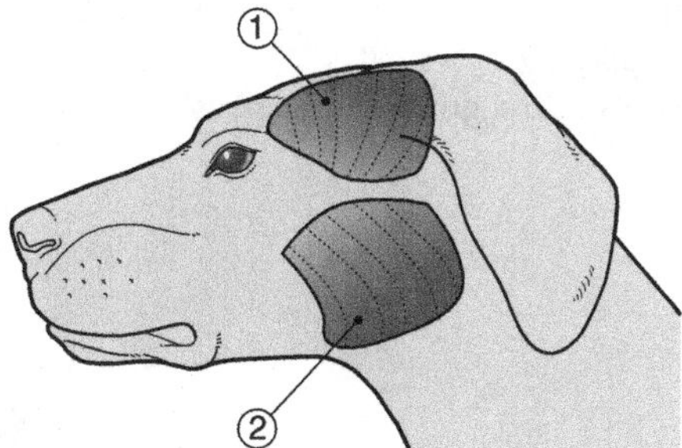

Figure 4.4 Drawing to create a jigsaw puzzle of an animal's head. 1. Temporal. 2. Masseter.

Activity

Below is a diagram of the muscles of the trunk and limbs. To make a jigsaw puzzle, follow the steps below.

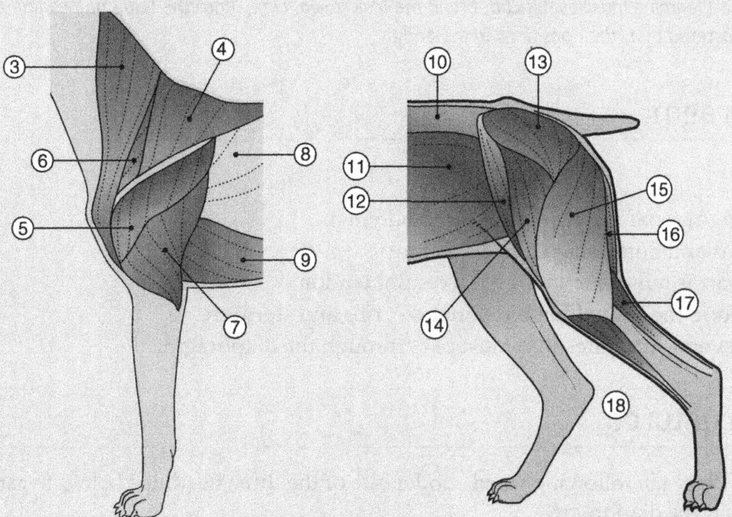

Figure 4.5 Drawing to create a jigsaw puzzle of an animal's trunk and limbs. 3. Brachiocephalicus. 4. Trapezius. 5. Deltod (trichoid). 6. Infraspinatous and supraspinatous. 7. Triceps brachii. 8. Latissimus dorsi. 9. Pectoral. 10. Lumbar epaxial. 11. Abdominal oblique. 12. Sartorius. 13. Gluteal. 14. Quadriceps femoris. 15. Biceps femoris. 16. Semitendinosis and semimembranosis. 17. Gastrocnemius. 18. Anterior tibialis. Note that the biceps brachii and brachialis are on the dorsomedial aspect of the elbow region.

1. Photocopy the diagram, enlarging it if necessary.
2. Colour in and label the photocopy.
3. Cut out each individual muscle.
4. Keep the pieces safe! You can use the pieces several times to help you learn muscular anatomy.

Mnemonic

To remember the muscles of the limbs.

Bef**ore** **t**rying **B**ritish **B**ulldog **p**laying,

I **s**at be**hind** **q**uiet **B**ichon **F**rise **s**niffing **g**reen **s**oggy **g**rass!

(Before) – the *fore*limb
Triceps
Biceps brachii
Pectoral
Infraspinatus
Supraspinatus
(Behind) – the *hind*limb
Quadriceps
Biceps femoris
Semitendinosus
Gluteal
Semimembranosus
Gastrocnemius

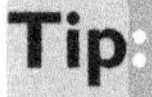

If you find learning muscles difficult, break the task down. First, learn the Latin names and then, when you have mastered that, their positions in the body.

The diaphragm

Key Points:

1. The diaphragm separates the thorax and abdomen.
2. It is flattened and dome shaped in appearance.
3. The outer part is muscular and it has a central tendon.
4. It is attached to the cranial lumbar vertebrae, ribs and sternum.
5. There are several structures that must pass through the diaphragm.

List the structures

Exercise 4.3 Place the following words under one of the three headings below to categorize their passage through the diaphragm.

(1)Aorta	(2)Oesophagus	(3)Caudal vena cava
(4)Vagus nerve	(5)Thoracic duct	(6)Azygos vein

Aortic hiatus	Oesophageal hiatus	Caval foramen

Tendons

Key Points:

1. Tendons are made of dense connective tissue.
2. They attach muscle to bone.

3. They should not be confused with ligaments, which attach bone to bone (except soft tissue ligaments as these support organs).
4. Tendons vary in shape depending on their position in the body and the type of muscle they are attached to.
5. Flat sheets of muscle tend to have flat tendons—these are called aponeuroses (sing. aponeurosis).
6. A sac (bursa) filled with synovial fluid is present where tendons pass over joints to reduce friction.

Link the words

Exercise 4.4 Match the description in the left-hand column to the correct definition in the right-hand column by drawing a line to link them.

(1)Tendon responsible for supporting caudal abdomen and aiding defaecation and parturition	(2)Linea alba
(3)Tendon inserting on the olecranon	(4)Prepubic tendon
(5)Aponeurosis of the abdominal midline	(6)Achilles tendon
(7)Tendon made up of the gastrocnemius, biceps femoris, semitendinosus and digital flexors	(8)Tendon of triceps brachii

Word chart

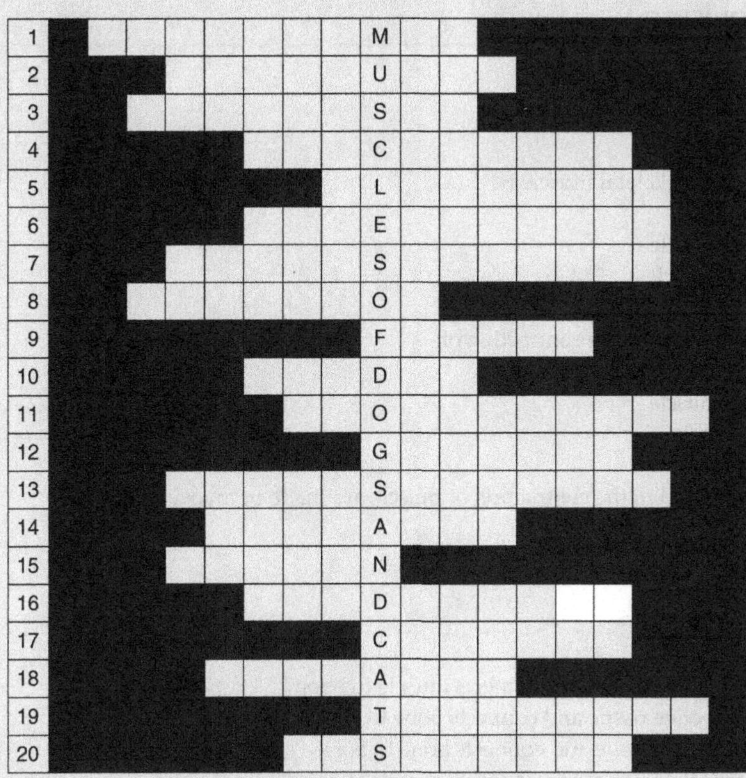

Exercise 4.5

1. First word of a flat muscle of the trunk that inserts on the humerus.
2. The term for one nerve fibre and the muscle fibres it innervates.
3. These muscles have finer movements and change the shapes of structures.
4. An elbow flexor found on the cranial forelimb.
5. Point of insertion of the triceps brachii.
6. Muscles found between the ribs, which play a role in respiration.
7. A shoulder extensor found in the supraspinous fossa.
8. The name for a muscle that increases the angle between bones.
9. The name for a muscle that decreases the angle between bones.
10. A structure that joins muscle to bone.
11. A flat sheet-like tendon.
12. Hip extensor and abductor muscles.
13. Large muscle found on the lateral thigh.
14. Another term for voluntary muscle.
15. The name of the tendon that is the most proximal or medial.
16. The tendon of this muscle contains the patella and inserts on the tibia.
17. The type of muscle that has pacemaker cells.
18. The second word of the muscle that lies on the cranial aspect of the tibia.
19. A flat muscle running from the cervical and thoracic vertebrae to the scapula.
20. The tendon that is more distal or lateral.

General revision

Multiple choice questions

Exercise 4.6

1. Another term for skeletal muscle is:
   a. cardiac muscle
   b. voluntary muscle
   c. unstriated muscle
   d. smooth muscle.
2. Peristalsis is the wave-like contraction of:
   a. cardiac muscle
   b. voluntary muscle
   c. striated muscle
   d. smooth muscle.
3. The fibres involved in the contraction of muscle are made of myosin and:
   a. haemoglobin
   b. pectin
   c. globulin
   d. actin.
4. A tendon is made of:
   a. loose connective tissue and connects muscle to bone
   b. dense connective tissue and connects bone to bone
   c. loose connective tissue and connects bone to bone
   d. dense connective tissue and connects muscle to bone.

5. A bursa which completely surrounds a tendon is called a:
   a. synovial joint
   b. sarcolemma
   c. synovial sheath
   d. sarcomere.

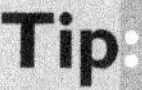

Why not get together with fellow students and write some more questions for each other?

What am I?

Exercise 4.7 Name the muscles described below, writing the correct answer in the space provided.

I lie on the lateral surface of the ramus of mandible and my action closes the mouth.	(1)
I am the largest muscle of the head and arise mainly from the parietal bone. My action closes the mouth.	(2)
I am a flat, wide muscle that lies on either side of the linea alba. My fibres run longitudinally.	(3)
A muscle of the thoracic limb, I arise on the scapula and cross the shoulder joint to insert on the cranial surface of the humerus. I am an elbow flexor and shoulder extensor.	(4)
I am a long muscle running from the ischial tuberosity to the mid-tibia on the caudal aspect. I am essentially an extensor but also play a part in foot placement and positioning.	(5)

CHAPTER 5

The nervous system and special senses

LEARNING **Objectives**

This chapter will help you to revise the following:

- facts and functions of the nervous system
- nerve tissue
- the central nervous system and related structures
- the peripheral nervous system
- reflexes
- facts and functions of the tongue
- the lingual papillae
- the sense of taste
- the sense of smell
- facts about the eye
- the structure and function of the eye
- structures surrounding the eye
- facts and functions of the ear
- the outer (external) ear
- the middle ear
- the inner ear
- the functions of the ear.

There is a general revision section at the end of the chapter.

THE NERVOUS SYSTEM

Facts and functions of the nervous system

1. The prefix denoting the nerves is *neur–*.
2. The nervous system has four main functions:
   a. to receive information from the internal environment, i.e. other systems of the body
   b. to receive information from the external environment, i.e. the animal's surroundings
   c. to interpret the information received
   d. to respond appropriately to the information received.
3. The nervous system has two main areas—the central nervous system and the peripheral nervous system.

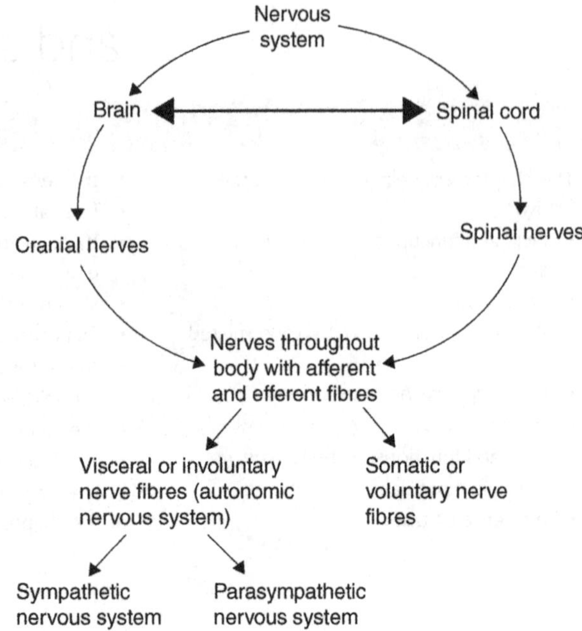

Figure 5.1 Diagram depicting the layout of the nervous system.

Activity

Assist with a neurological examination of a cat or dog. Observe the animal's responses to the various stimuli and consider what is actually happening in the nervous system.

Nerve tissue

Key Points:

1. Like other body tissues, nerve tissue is made up of cells. Nerve cells are called *neurons*.
2. Neurons form a vast communication network throughout the animal body by using a system of impulses.
3. Nerve impulses move from one neuron to another to send 'messages' to various parts of the body.
4. Nerve fibres are the long fine axons of the cell extending from the cell body.
5. Nerves are bundles of nerve fibres held together in a connective tissue sheath.
6. Sensory or afferent nerve fibres *receive* information from the peripheral nervous system and take it to the central nervous system.
7. Motor or efferent nerve fibres *send* information from the central nervous system to the peripheral nervous system.
8. A nerve may be made up of sensory, motor, or both sensory and motor fibres.
9. Grey matter is the term used to describe the appearance of cell bodies.
10. White matter is the term used to describe the appearance of axons or fibres.

Activity

Exercise 5.1 Below is a diagram of a neuron. From the selection, add the correct labels.

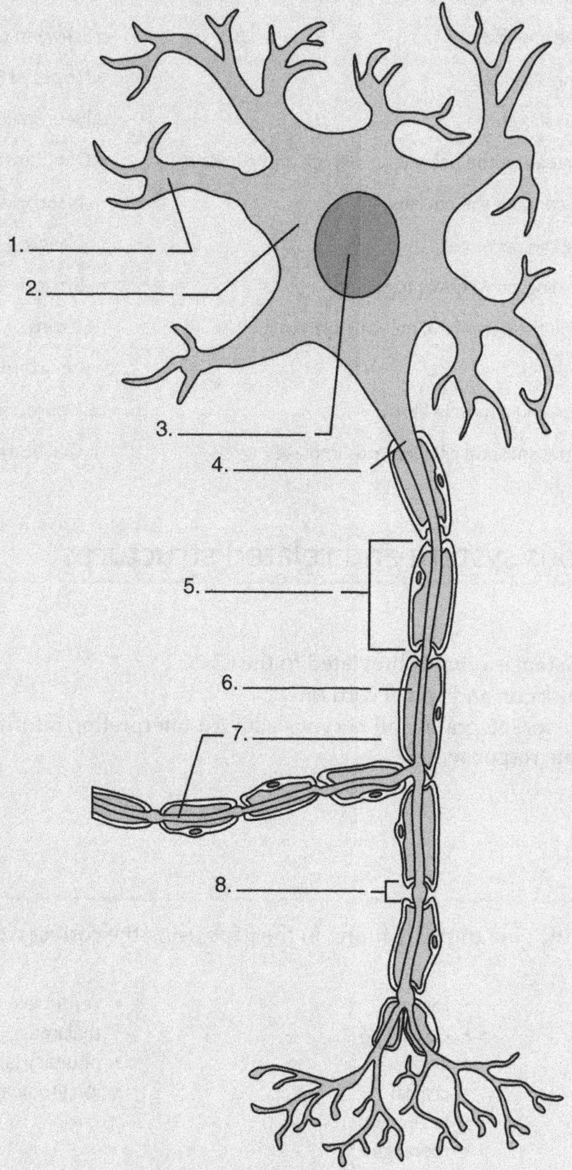

Nucleus	Schwann cell	Node of Ranvier	Cell body
Myelin sheath	Dendrite	Axon	Axon branch (collateral axon)

Figure 5.2 Diagram of a neuron.

(Reproduced with kind permission from Colville & Bassert 2002.)

Link the words

Exercise 5.2 Match the description in the left-hand column to the correct definition in the right-hand column by drawing a line to link them.

(1)Short projections that receive impulses	(2)Schwann cells
(3)Long projections that transmit impulses	(4)Nodes of Ranvier
(5)Cells that produce the myelin sheath	(6)Neuromuscular junction
(7)Gaps in the myelin sheath that allow the passage of oxygen and nutrients	(8)Dendrites
(9)The part of the neuron that contains the nucleus	(10)Neuroglia
(11)The membrane surrounding the nerve cell	(12)Ganglion
(13)Dense connective tissue holding nerve fibres together	(14)Synapse
(15)Group of cell bodies found in the peripheral nervous system	(16)Axons
(17)The space between two neurons	(18)Neurilemma
(19)The space between a neuron and a muscle fibre	(20)Neurotransmitter
(21)A chemical that allows the transmission of a nervous impulse	(22)Cell body

The central nervous system and related structures

Key Points:

1. The central nervous system is often abbreviated to the CNS.
2. The CNS comprises the brain and spinal cord only.
3. The CNS is responsible for integrating all nervous activity, interpreting information and initiating an appropriate response.

Fill in the gaps

Exercise 5.3 Complete the paragraph by filling in the gaps using the correct words from the selection below.

- cerebrospinal fluid
- hypothalamus
- cardiovascular
- cerebellum
- temperature control
- pons
- four
- cerebrum
- two
- cranial
- brainstem
- meninges
- ventricles
- thalamus
- pituitary gland
- longitudinal sulcus

The main 'control centre' of the body, the brain is found in the (1)__________ cavity surrounded by three layers of protective membrane called the (2)__________. There are (3)__________chambers in the brain called the (4)__________ where (5)__________ is produced. The (6)__________is the large mass overlying the rest of the brain and is separated into (7)__________ hemispheres by the (8)__________. It receives, processes and stores information from all over the body. The (9)__________ is a paired structure that lies deep within each cerebral hemisphere and acts as a relay station for information. Lying beneath this is the (10)__________, which is responsible for basic physiological functions such as hunger,

(11)__________ and sexual drive. It is also a major link with the endocrine system and controls the secretions of the (12)__________, which lies directly beneath it. The caudal region of the brain is the (13)__________, which co-ordinates muscular activity. The (14)__________ and medulla oblongata are found in the ventrocaudal area where the spinal cord attaches to the brain. This area is also known as the (15)__________. The medulla oblongata contains a centre responsible for governing the respiratory and (16)__________ systems.

Tip: *The brain is sometimes divided into three sections—the fore-, mid- and hindbrain. This is anatomically convenient but bears no reference to the functions of the various parts of the brain.*

Table 5.1 The anatomically convenient sections of the brain

Forebrain	Midbrain	Hindbrain
Cerebrum	Relay stations between different structures	Pons
Thalamus		Cerebllum
Hypothalamus		Medulla oblongata

The spinal cord

Facts about the spinal cord:

1. The spinal cord integrates and relays information from all areas of the nervous system.
2. The spinal cord runs down the centre of the vertebral column, in the vertebral foramen.
3. The spinal cord enters the cranial cavity via the foramen magnum and attaches to the brainstem.
4. The spinal cord terminates at the last few lumbar vertebrae where it gradually separates into a series of nerves; the effect resembles a horse's tail and is called the *cauda equina.*
5. The spinal cord is surrounded by three protective membranes, the meninges.
6. At each intervertebral space, a pair of spinal nerves leaves the spinal cord.

Activity

Exercise 5.4 Below is a diagram of a spinal cord. From the selection, add the correct labels.

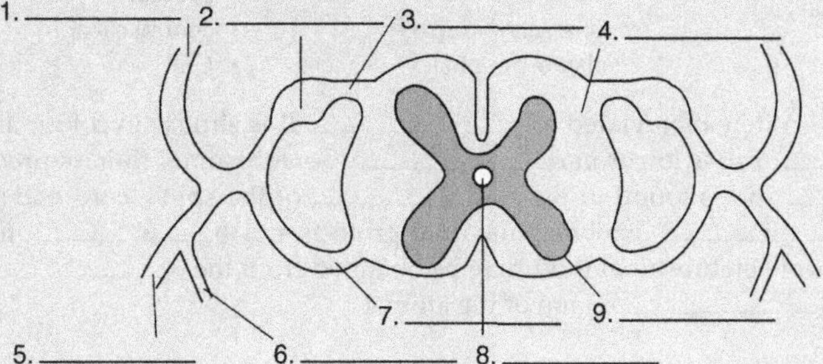

Dorsal root	Grey matter	Ventral root	Nerve to epaxial region	To sympathetic chain
White matter	Nerve to hypaxial muscles, body wall and limbs	Central canal	Dorsal root ganglion	

Figure 5.3 Diagram of a section through the spinal cord.
(Reproduced with kind permission from Lane & Cooper 1999.)

The meninges

The meninges are three concentric protective membranes surrounding the brain and spinal cord.

Activity

Exercise 5.5 Fill in the table so that each column contains three facts from the selection below.

(1) The inner membrane

(2) Space below is filled with cerebrospinal fluid: the subarachnoid space

(3) Not closely connected in the vertebral column to form the epidural space

(4) A vascular membrane

(5) A web-like membrane

(6) The outer membrane

(7) Closely follows the contours of the brain

(8) The middle membrane

(9) A tough fibrous membrane

Dura mater	Arachnoid mater	Pia mater

Fill in the gaps

Exercise 5.6 Complete the paragraph on cerebrospinal fluid by filling in the gaps using the correct words from the selection below.

- blood plasma
- cushions
- protein
- ventricles
- subarachnoid space
- central canal
- cisterna magna
- atlanto-occipital
- CSF

Cerebrospinal fluid is often abbreviated to (1)__________. It is similar in colour and composition to (2)__________ but is lower in (3)__________. Cerebrospinal fluid is produced in the brain (4)__________ and is found in the (5)__________ of the spinal cord and surrounding the CNS in the (6)__________. Cerebrospinal fluid protects and (7)__________ the brain and spinal cord. Samples of cerebrospinal fluid may be obtained from the (8)__________ by inserting a needle in the (9)__________ region of the animal.

The peripheral nervous system

Key Points:

1. The peripheral nervous system comprises all parts of the nervous system except the brain and spinal cord (CNS).

2. The peripheral nervous system is often abbreviated to PNS.
3. The PNS is made up of a network of nerves with afferent (sensory) and efferent (motor) fibres, which serve all areas of the body. These nerves eventually connect to the CNS via either the spinal nerves or the cranial nerves.
4. *Somatic nerves* serve voluntary parts of the body.
5. *Visceral nerves* serve involuntary parts of the body.
6. The involuntary nerves are often termed the autonomic nervous system (ANS) and are referred to as a discrete section of the nervous system. (Some texts term just the efferent visceral nerves the ANS.)

The spinal and cranial nerves

Most nerves of the PNS enter or leave the CNS via the spinal nerves, which exit the spinal cord at each intervertebral space. However, there are 12 pairs of nerves that arise directly from the ventral surface of the brain. All but one pair serve functions purely in the head and neck.

Link the words

Exercise 5.7 Match the cranial nerve in the left-hand column to the correct function in the right-hand column by drawing a line to link them.

(1)I. Olfactory	(2)Jaw muscles
(3)II. Optic	(4)Hearing and balance
(5)III. Oculomotor	(6)Eye muscles
(7)IV. Trochlear	(8)Mouth and pharynx
(9)V. Trigeminal	(10)Pharynx, larynx, neck, thorax and abdomen
(11)VI. Abducens	(12)Eye muscles
(13)VII. Facial	(14)Vision
(15)VIII. Vestibulocochlear	(16)Neck
(17)IX. Glossopharyngeal	(18)Smell
(19)X. Vagus	(20)Facial expression
(21)XI. Accessory	(22)Tongue
(23)XII. Hypoglossal	(24)Eye muscles

Mnemonic

To remember the cranial nerves.

Oh! Oh! Oh! To try and find very godly vicars around here!

The autonomic nervous system

This is another term for the visceral (involuntary) nerves of the PNS. The autonomic nervous system (ANS) is separated into two sections with opposing effects.

Look it up

Exercise 5.8 Fill in the table to show the effect each part of the ANS has on the body functions or parts listed.

	Sympathetic	Parasympathetic
Heart rate	(1)	(2)
Respiratory rate	(3)	(4)
Blood vessels	(5)	(6)
Intestinal movement	(7)	(8)
Pupils	(9)	(10)

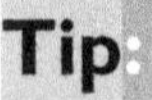

The sympathetic part of the ANS prepares the body for action ('fight or flight'). Remember that 'S' stands for 'stress' to help you remember its action!

Reflexes

Key Points:

1. A reflex is a fixed involuntary response to certain stimuli.
2. The simplest form of reflex is a spinal reflex but other reflexes can involve areas of the brain called reflex centres.
3. Spinal reflexes involve the PNS and spinal cord alone and do not involve the brain.

Activity

Design a poster on A3 paper depicting a diagram of the nerve activity that occurs when a dog stands on a sharp thorn. Add the following labels:

- afferent (sensory) nerve pathway
- efferent (motor) nerve pathway
- dorsal root of spinal nerve
- ventral root of spinal nerve
- intercalating neuron.

Use large labels and bold colours. When it is complete, stick it where you will regularly read it. Why not on a kitchen cupboard?

Study

In animals, spinal cord activity exceeds cerebral activity, indicating that animals rely heavily on reflexes. List as many reflexes as you can and consider which part of the CNS is involved. Is it a spinal or a cerebral reflex?

THE TONGUE, TASTE AND SMELL

Facts and functions of the tongue

1. The tongue is made up of two sections—the body and the root. The term *lingual* pertains to the tongue.
2. The body of the tongue is connected to the ventral surface of the oral cavity by the lingual frenulum, although its root is in the pharynx.
3. The tongue is mostly made of skeletal muscle covered with stratified squamous epithelium.
4. The tongue is served by cranial nerves V, VII, IX and XII.
5. The dorsal surface of the tongue has a groove running down its centre (the *median sulcus*) and a rough texture due to keratinization and the presence of a number of *papillae*, which are small projections arising from the tongue's surface.
6. Papillae may contain serous glands, mucous glands or taste buds, or a combination of two or more of these structures.
7. The paired lingual vein and artery run along the ventral surface of the tongue.

Link the words

Exercise 5.9 Match the description in the left-hand column to the correct definition in the right-hand column by drawing a line to link them.

(1)Panting to cool down	(2)Lapping
(3)The sense of taste	(4)Prehension
(5)Excessively long and cornified papillae in the cat are for this purpose	(6)Manipulation of food
(7)The animal must move the food bolus to the pharynx in order to swallow	(8)Evaporative heat loss
(9)Both dogs and cats drink in this way	(10)Mechanical digestion
(11)Food begins to be broken down by the teeth and tongue	(12)Grooming
(13)Some types of food can be taken into the mouth with the aid of the tongue	(14)Gustation

The lingual papillae

Key Points:

1. A papilla is a dome-shaped protuberance.
2. Several different types of papillae occur on the dorsal surface of the tongue:
   a. filiform papillae; these are the smallest and most numerous. They are serrated in shape and appear on the more rostral two-thirds of the dorsal surface. Their function is mainly tactile or sensory. It is these papillae that are well developed to facilitate grooming in cats
   b. fungiform papillae; these are mushroom-shaped papillae, which appear on the more rostral two-thirds of the dorsal surface. Their main function is gustation
   c. foliate papillae; these have a mainly gustatory function and appear on the more caudal third of the dorsolateral surface
   d. conical papillae; also situated on the more caudal third, these circular papillae are mainly tactile or sensory

e. vallate (or circumvallate) papillae; there are 3 to 6 of these mainly gustatory papillae in a V-shape (pointing caudally) situated on the more caudal third of the dorsal surface
f. marginal papillae; these are seen on the rostral tongue margins of unweaned young. They create a vacuum seal useful for suckling milk and disappear as soon as the animal begins a solid diet.

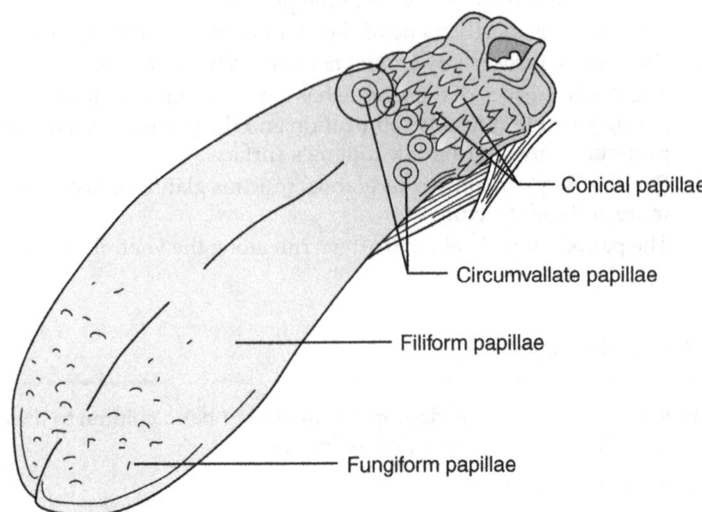

Figure 5.4 Diagram of the position of papillae on the tongue. (Adapted with permission from Colville & Bassert 2002.)

The sense of taste

Key Points:

1. Taste (gustation) is possible due to the presence of taste buds.
2. Taste buds are found in many of the papillae on the dorsal surface of the tongue.
3. Within the taste buds are taste cells; these are specialized chemoreceptors for detecting water-soluble chemicals.
4. There are four tastes detectable to dogs—salt, sour, bitter and sweet, and three tastes detectable to cats—salt, sour and bitter. All other tastes are a combination of these together with information gained by olfaction.
5. Different areas on the tongue are sensitive to different tastes; whilst sour and bitter are detectable across the tongue surface, salt is only detectable on the rostral two-thirds, and sweet only at the tip.

The sense of smell

Key Points:

1. Smell (olfaction) is a highly developed sense in both cats and dogs.
2. The main organ of olfaction is Jacobson's organ (or the vomeronasal organ), which is a paired sac situated at the rostral base of the nasal septum.

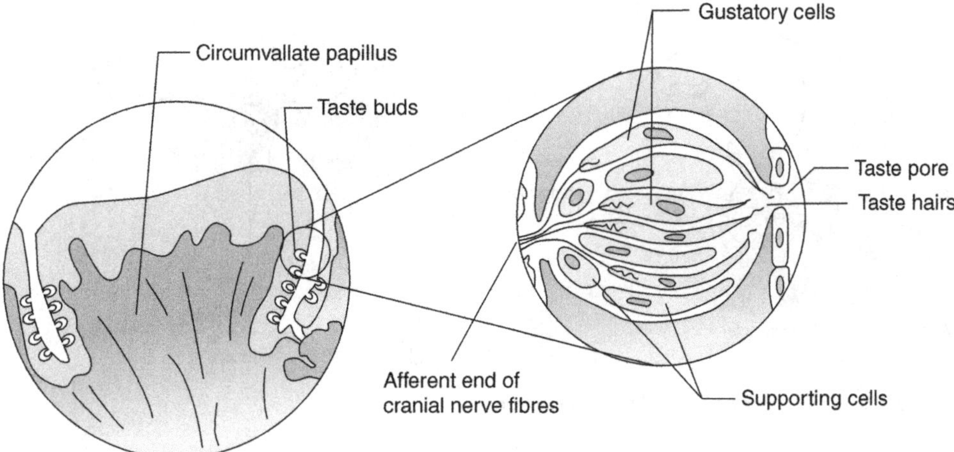

Figure 5.5 Diagram of a taste bud.
(Adapted with permission from Colville & Bassert 2002.)

3. The vomeronasal organ is made up of specialized chemoreceptor cells for detecting airborne chemicals.
4. There are also some olfactory chemoreceptors in the lining of the nasal cavity.
5. Unlike gustation, where there are only four main taste types, there are hundreds of smells detectable by dogs and cats.
6. Gustation and olfaction often work in conjunction to heighten an animal's awareness of its environment, especially during food selection.
7. As well as air inhaled through the nares, a dog or cat may detect smells from the oral cavity via two tiny ducts called incisive ducts.
8. The incisive ducts run through the hard palate to connect the oral and nasal cavities; their use is also important in pheromone detection, when male animals will make rapid licking movements, or curl their upper lip to take in air. This is called the olfactory reflex or 'flehmen'.

THE EYE

Facts about the eye

1. The organ of vision—the eye—is a highly specialized organ, enabling images to be focused and detected by light-sensitive cells called photoreceptors.
2. The eye is formed from part of the forebrain in the ectodermal layer of the developing fetus.
3. Dogs and cats are born with their eyelid margins sealed together. They separate at approximately 10 to 14 days of age, although the retina is not fully formed until 6 weeks after birth.
4. In common with other predators, dogs and cats have forward-facing eyes. Although this restricts the sideways field of vision, it does mean that vision is mainly binocular, rather than the mainly monocular field seen by grazing animals. Binocular vision provides a greater perception of depth and distance, which is vital for hunting prey.
5. Eye structure is adapted to suit species lifestyle. For example, the cornea of the nocturnal cat is larger, relatively speaking, than the cornea of the diurnal dog. This allows for the maximum penetration of light rays.
6. The prefix denoting the eye is *ophthalm–*.

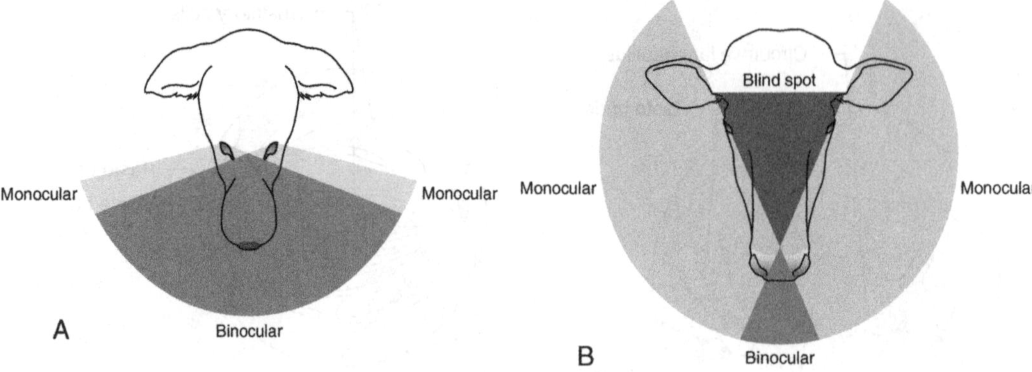

Figure 5.6 Diagram of monocular and binocular vision.

The structure and function of the eye

Key Points:

1. The eyeball (or globe) is made up of three distinct layers (tunics):
   a. the outer protective layer (sclera)
   b. the middle vascular layer (choroid)
   c. the inner nervous layer (retina).
2. These layers are interrupted at the front of the eye where the anatomy is adapted to allow for the entrance of light and focusing. The globe also bulges outwards in this area.
3. Inside the globe, there are three chambers:
   a. the anterior chamber between the cornea and the iris
   b. the posterior chamber between the iris and the lens
   c. the vitreous chamber behind the lens.
4. The anterior and posterior chambers are filled with a jelly-like fluid called aqueous humour.
5. The vitreous chamber is filled with jelly-like vitreous humour.
6. The functions of the humours are:
   a. to provide nutrients
   b. to remove waste products
   c. to maintain the shape and pressure of the globe to allow consistent light refraction.
7. The amount of light allowed into the vitreous chamber is determined by pupil size, which is controlled by the muscles of the iris.
8. The refraction of light and the focusing of an image onto the retina occur in three places:
   a. as light travels through the transparent cornea
   b. as light moves through the aqueous and vitreous humours
   c. as light moves through the lens, which changes shape by contraction or relaxation of the muscular ciliary body.
9. Light stimulates the photoreceptor cells in the retina, which causes impulses to be sent from neighbouring bipolar receptor cells along the optic nerve.
10. There are two main types of photoreceptor cell:
    a. rods, which are associated with black and white vision
    b. cones, which are associated with colour vision.
11. The retina of the dog and cat comprises mainly rods, although there are some cones present. Although they can differentiate some colours, they cannot distinguish subtle shade differences;

this is known as dichromatic vision. (Humans and some other primates have trichromatic vision.)

12. The optic nerves from each eye cross at the optic chiasma on the ventral surface of the brain before entering the cerebral cortex via the midbrain.

Activity

Exercise 5.10 Below is a diagram of a mammalian eye. From the selection, add the correct labels.

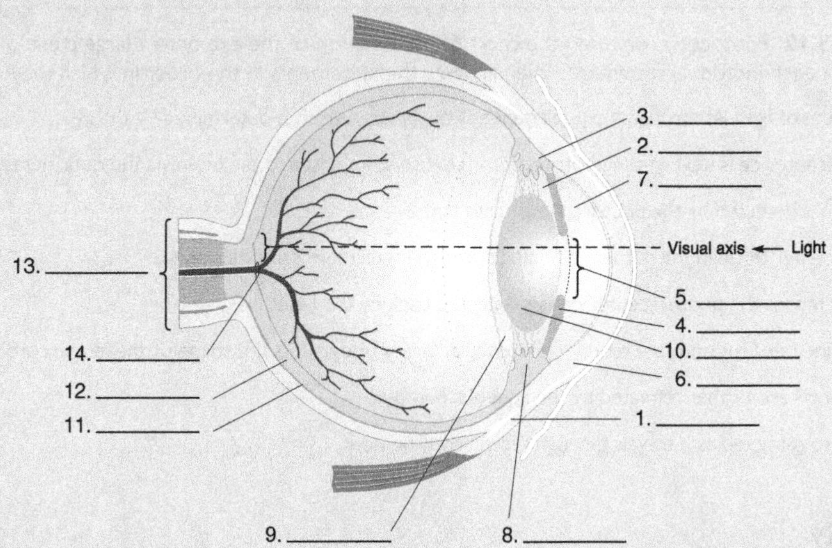

Sclera	Cornea	Optic nerve	Limbus	Posterior chamber
Lens	Optic disc	Suspensory ligaments	Iris	Pupil
Choroid	Retina	Ciliary body	Anterior chamber	

Figure 5.7 Diagram of the eye.
(Reproduced with kind permission from Colville & Bassert 2002.)

Link the words

Exercise 5.11 Match the description in the left-hand column to the correct definition in the right-hand column by drawing a line to link them.

(1)The vascular layer of the globe	(2)Optic disc
(3)The collective name for the choroid, iris and ciliary body	(4)Pupil
(5)The convex structure that focuses light rays onto the retina	(6)Choroid
(7)The transparent surface at the front of the eye through which light rays pass	(8)Rods and cones

(Continued)

(9)The 'blind spot' on the retina	(10)Uvea
(11)The shiny inner surface of the choroid	(12)Lens
(13)Photosensitive cells	(14)Sclera
(15)The hole in the centre of the iris	(16)Cornea
(17)The white, fibrous protective layer of the globe	(18)Tapetum

Activity

Exercise 5.12 Photocopy (or copy) the chart of the function of the eye onto a large piece of paper and cut out each individual statement. Then arrange the statements in the order in which they occur.

(1)The amount of light let through the pupil depends on its size, which is determined by the iris.

(2)Bipolar receptor cells next to the photoreceptor cells send impulses to the brain via the optic nerve.

(3)The image is detected by the photoreceptor cells in the retina.

(4)Light rays enter through the cornea. Its shape starts to focus them onto the retina.

(5)Light that misses the photoreceptor cells is reflected back by the tapetum.

(6)The lens focuses light onto the retina. The muscular ciliary body alters the shape of the lens accordingly.

(7)The light rays are further refracted by the aqueous humour.

(8)Light is also refracted as it travels through the vitreous humour.

Activity

Take the opportunity to examine an animal's eye using an ophthalmoscope. Ask for help to identify the structures you see.

Structures surrounding the eye

Key Points:

1. Known as the adnexa, the structures surrounding the eye include the following:
   a. orbit and surrounding bone
   b. muscles
   c. conjunctiva
   d. eyelids
   e. eyelashes
   f. lacrimal apparatus.
2. The eye socket (or orbit) houses the globe, a cushioning fat pad and surrounding musculature. Bones bordering the orbit are the:
   a. maxilla
   b. frontal bone
   c. zygomatic arch
   d. lacrimal bone
   e. sphenoid bone.

3. Muscles allow movement of the globe as follows:
   a. the medial, lateral, dorsal and ventral rectus muscles allow movement up, down and left to right, respectively
   b. the retractor oculi muscle allows slight retraction of the globe into the orbit
   c. the dorsal and ventral oblique muscles allow slight rotation
   d. the palpebral muscles are the muscles of the eyelids.
4. The eyelids, or palpebrae (singular, palpebra), comprise a fibrous layer (the tarsal plate) covered with skin and mucous membrane, which continues to line the eye as conjunctiva. The pocket formed between the conjunctiva and the globe is called the *fornix*.
5. The upper and lower palpebrae meet in the corners of the eyes; these are the medial canthus and the lateral canthus.
6. Meibomian glands in the palpebrae produce a fatty secretion that forms around 10% of tear film.
7. The third eyelid (or nictitating membrane) contains cartilage and is covered on both sides by mucous membrane and lymph nodules. A pear-shaped gland that contributes to tear film is also found in the third eyelid.
8. Known as cilia, the eyelashes of dogs line the edge of the lid and protect the globe. Carnivores, including cats, do not have true eyelashes.
9. The main lacrimal gland lies by the dorsolateral wall of the orbit. Its production, lacrimal fluid, which makes up the bulk of tear film, lubricates and protects the eye and maintains the transparency of the cornea.
10. Lacrimal fluid drains into the lacrimal punctae (singular, puncta), or tear ducts, which are found on both eyelids at the medial canthus of each eye. The tear ducts drain into the nasolacrimal duct, which empties into the nasal cavity.

Study

For each of the eye diseases listed below, describe the meaning, breeds commonly affected and common treatment methods.

Disease	Description	Breeds affected	Treatment
Distichiasis			
Keratoconjunctivitis sicca			
Entropion			
Ectropion			

THE EAR

Facts and functions of the ear

1. The ear is the organ of hearing and balance.
2. The term *aural* relates to the ear.
3. The prefix denoting the ear is *ot–*.
4. The prefix denoting hearing is *audi–*.
5. Hearing is usually functional at around 14 days of age.

The outer (external) ear

Key Points:

1. The outer ear comprises the pinna (ear flap) and auditory canal, which is separated into vertical and horizontal sections.
2. The pinna is a flat cartilage (the *auricular cartilage*) covered on both sides by skin.
3. The shape of the pinna is determined by breed in the dog, although cats' pinnae tend to look more similar in shape, being triangular, forward facing and erect.
4. The outer surface of the pinna is usually covered in hair, but hair on the inner surface tends to be sparser in most breeds.
5. A cutaneous pouch or pocket is found on the lateral border of each pinna in both dogs and cats.
6. Several muscles attach to the auricular cartilage, which makes each pinna highly mobile and able to be directed towards sound for optimum sound wave collection.
7. Once collected, sound waves are channelled into the auditory canal, a tube lined with specialized skin, which is supported by another small cartilage (the *annular cartilage*).
8. The skin of the auditory canal contains specialized sebaceous glands (ceruminous glands), which produce *cerumen* (earwax).
9. The horizontal part of the canal runs into a hole in the temporal bone (the external acoustic meatus) to meet the tympanic membrane.

Activity

Exercise 5.13 Below is a diagram of the external ear. From the selection, add the correct labels.

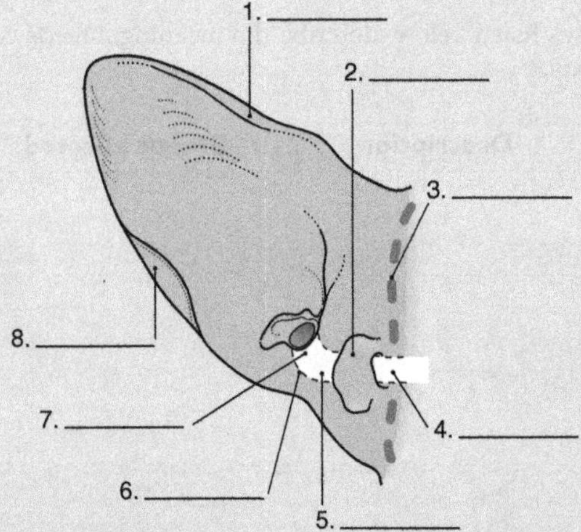

Auditory canal (horizontal section)	Auricular cartilage covered with skin	Marginal cutaneous pouch	Auditory canal (vertical section)
Annular cartilage surrounding canal	External acoustic meatus	Specialized skin containing ceruminous glands	Temporal bone

Figure 5.8 Diagram of the outer ear.
(Adapted with kind permission from Evans 1993.)

Activity

Take every opportunity to examine the ears of dogs and cats both with the naked eye and using an auriscope to learn the structural appearance of normal and abnormal outer ears.
Which breeds commonly have ear disease? Consider why this could be. Note the different pinna shapes, the amount of cerumen present and the amount of hair on the inner surface of the pinna, which may even extend down into the ear canal.

The middle ear

Key Points:

1. The middle ear begins at the tympanic membrane (ear drum), which is a thin oval membrane made of connective tissue and stratified squamous epithelium.
2. The middle ear (tympanic cavity) is an air-filled space housed in the tympanic bulla of the skull.
3. Running across the tympanic cavity are three small bones known as auditory ossicles:
   a. the malleus (hammer)
   b. the incus (anvil)
   c. the stapes (stirrup).
4. The malleus attaches to the inner surface of the tympanic membrane and the stapes attaches to one of the membranes separating the middle and inner parts of the ear; this is the vestibular (oval) window. The incus sits between the two, forming a link across the tympanic cavity.
5. A tube running from the tympanic cavity to the nasopharynx provides an external opening to enable air pressure to remain equal either side of the tympanic membrane. This is known as the auditory or Eustachian tube.
6. Below the vestibular window there is another small membrane between the middle and inner parts of the ear called the cochlear (round) window.

Activity

Think about how the auditory tube works. To help you, consider what happens when you take off in an aeroplane or dive deeply in a swimming pool. How does the change in external pressure affect you and what do you do to remedy the situation?

The inner ear

Key Points:

1. Inside the temporal bone is a fluid-filled cavity known as the bony labyrinth. Inside this bony labyrinth is a series of fluid-filled chambers and tubes, which are all interconnected and known as the membranous labyrinth.

2. The fluid inside the bony labyrinth surrounding the membranous labyrinth is known as perilymph.
3. The fluid inside the membranous labyrinth is known as endolymph.
4. Inside the membranous labyrinth are the organs of hearing and balance.
5. Parallel with the cochlear window is a small coiled structure resembling a snail's shell; this is the cochlea, which is around 7 mm high. Inside the cochlea runs a duct filled with endolymph, which reaches it via a small sac (the saccule).
6. At the end of the coiled cochlea is a sensory area known as the organ of Corti, which has a close association with cranial nerve VIII.
7. Parallel with the vestibular window is a chamber known as the utricle. Arising from the utricle are three endolymph-filled semicircular canals that sit at right-angles to each other.
8. Each semicircular canal is about 0.5 mm in diameter and has a bulge (ampulla) at its base.
9. Lining the ampulla are sensory hairs called crista.
10. The utricle and saccule are joined together creating a link between the semicircular canals and the cochlea. Both contain further sensory areas called maculae.
11. Endolymph fills the membranous labyrinth from a small sac in the subarachnoid space via the endolymphatic duct.

Link the words

Exercise 5.14 Match the description in the left-hand column to the correct definition in the right-hand column by drawing a line to link them.

(1)The fluid surrounding the membranous labyrinth	(2)Ampulla
(3)The sensory area in the cochlea	(4)Maculae
(5)The small sac joining the cochlea and the utricle	(6)Crista
(7)The bulge at the base of a semicircular canal	(8)Perilymph
(9)Sensory hairs in the ampulla	(10)Endolymph
(11)The fluid inside the membranous labyrinth	(12)Organ of Corti
(13)Sensory areas found in the utricle and saccule	(14)Saccule
(15)The base of the semicircular canals	(16)Utricle

The functions of the ear

Key Points:

1. The two functions of the ear are hearing and balance.
2. The sensory organs are all contained within the inner ear; the other sections of the ear collect and amplify sound waves.
3. The close connection between the organs of hearing and balance mean that when one part is diseased, the other is often affected. This is seen in cases of otitis interna.

Fill in the gaps

Exercise 5.15 Complete the paragraph on hearing and balance by filling in the gaps using the correct words from the selection below.

- saccule
- maculae
- crista
- tympanic
- utricle
- ossicles
- pinna
- cochlear
- vestibulocochlear
- semicircular
- Corti
- endolymph

Hearing

Sound waves are channelled towards the auditory canal by the (1)__________, which can change shape and direction. The sound waves pass through the (2)__________ membrane and across the middle ear via the auditory (3)__________. Once into the inner ear, the waves move through the endolymph in the (4)__________ duct to be detected by the organ of (5)__________, which contains sensory hairs. These hairs react to different frequencies, and impulses are then sent to the brain via cranial nerve VIII, the (6)__________ nerve.

Balance

In the inner ear, three mutually perpendicular (7)__________ canals are situated. As (8)__________ moves to and fro in the canals, sensory (9)__________ detect the direction of the movement and transmit impulses to cranial nerve VIII. The semicircular canals join together at a base called the (10)__________. Further down, towards the cochlea, is another sac, the (11)__________. Both the utricle and the saccule contain sensory (12)__________, which detect orientation.

General revision

Multiple choice questions – the nervous system

Exercise 5.16

1. The gap between two neurons is called a:
   a. neurilemma
   b. synapse
   c. axon
   d. neuroglia.
2. The gap between a neuron and a muscle fibre is called a:
   a. node of Ranvier
   b. myelin sheath
   c. neuromuscular junction
   d. epidural space.
3. A collection of cell bodies lying outside the CNS is called a:
   a. ganglion
   b. dendrite
   c. nucleus
   d. neuron.
4. Acetylcholine and noradrenaline are both chemicals found in synapses. Their function is
   a. neurotransmission
   b. the passage of oxygen
   c. the removal of waste
   d. the production of myelin.

5. An impulse reaches the CNS from the PNS via the:
   a. afferent nerves
   b. brain
   c. efferent nerves
   d. spinal cord.
6. Cranial nerve VII is the:
   a. optic
   b. hypoglossal
   c. abducens
   d. facial.
7. The cranial nerve which serves a function in the thorax is the:
   a. olfactory
   b. vestibulocochlear
   c. vagus
   d. trigeminal.
8. The sensory pathway of a spinal reflex enters the spinal cord via the:
   a. cranial nerves
   b. dorsal root
   c. intercalating neuron
   d. ventral root.

Tip *Why not get together with fellow students and write some more questions for each other?*

Study

Exercise 5.17 For each of the following, list the nervous system involvement in the order in which it would take place, for example:

Dog sees playmates in the park

- sensory (afferent) pathway via cranial nerve sends information to the brain
- brain interprets information
- motor (efferent) pathway via spinal nerves sends information to skeletal muscles to move dog in direction of playmates.

Try these:

— *Dog steps on a shard of glass while running*
— *Dog reaches playmates but is distracted by the smell of a nearby butcher's shop*
— *Dog reaches shop and tries to enter but the butcher throws a bucket of cold water over the dog!*
— *Dog's paw starts to hurt and he limps off in direction of home.*

Multiple choice questions – the tongue, taste and smell

Exercise 5.18

1. The lingual frenulum is:
   a. the keratinized mucous membrane on the dorsal surface of the tongue
   b. the border of the tongue margins where keratinized skin becomes non-keratinized skin
   c. a fold of mucous membrane running between the tongue and the ventral surface of the oral cavity
   d. the collective term for the voluntary muscle of the tongue.

2. The tongue is served by cranial nerves:
   a. V, VII, IX and XII
   b. V, VIII, X and XI
   c. IV, V, IX and X
   d. III, V, IX and XII.
3. The foliate papillae are found on the:
   a. rostral third of the tongue
   b. rostral two-thirds of the tongue
   c. caudal third of the tongue
   d. caudal two-thirds of the tongue.
4. Taste buds contain:
   a. photoreceptors
   b. mechanoreceptors
   c. electroreceptors
   d. chemoreceptors.
5. The key organ of olfaction is the:
   a. tongue
   b. nasal septum
   c. vomeronasal organ
   d. vallate papillae.

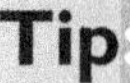

Why not get together with fellow students and write some more questions for each other?

Multiple choice questions – the eye

Exercise 5.19

1. Intraocular muscles:
   a. alter retinal shape
   b. regulate pupil size and lens shape
   c. cause the production of aqueous humour
   d. detect light rays.
2. Dorsal and ventral oblique muscles allow:
   a. dorsoventral movement of the globe
   b. retraction of the globe
   c. closing of the palpebrae
   d. rotation of the globe.
3. The middle vascular layer of the globe, which incorporates the choroid, iris and ciliary body, is the:
   a. fornix
   b. conjunctiva
   c. uvea
   d. chiasma.
4. The terminal part of the optic nerve is known as the 'blind spot' or:
   a. optic disc
   b. pupil
   c. lens
   d. lacrimal puncta.
5. The structure responsible for reflecting light back onto the retina is the:
   a. iris
   b. tapetum

c. cornea
d. sclera.

6. The lens is connected to the ciliary body by the:
   a. iris
   b. suspensory ligaments
   c. rectus muscles
   d. limbus.
7. The lacrimal punctae are found on:
   a. the upper eyelids at the lateral canthus only
   b. the lower eyelids at the medial canthus only
   c. both eyelids at the lateral canthus
   d. both eyelids at the medial canthus.
8. The pupils of the cat are:
   a. horizontal and elliptical
   b. circular
   c. rectangular
   d. vertical and elliptical.
9. 'Cones' are:
   a. photosensitive cells associated with black and white vision
   b. nerve fibres in the optic nerve
   c. photosensitive cells associated with colour vision
   d. bipolar receptor cells found alongside photoreceptor cells.
10. The cornea is a continuation of the:
    a. tapetum
    b. sclera
    c. choroid
    d. retina.

Tip: *Why not get together with fellow students and write some more questions for each other?*

Crossword

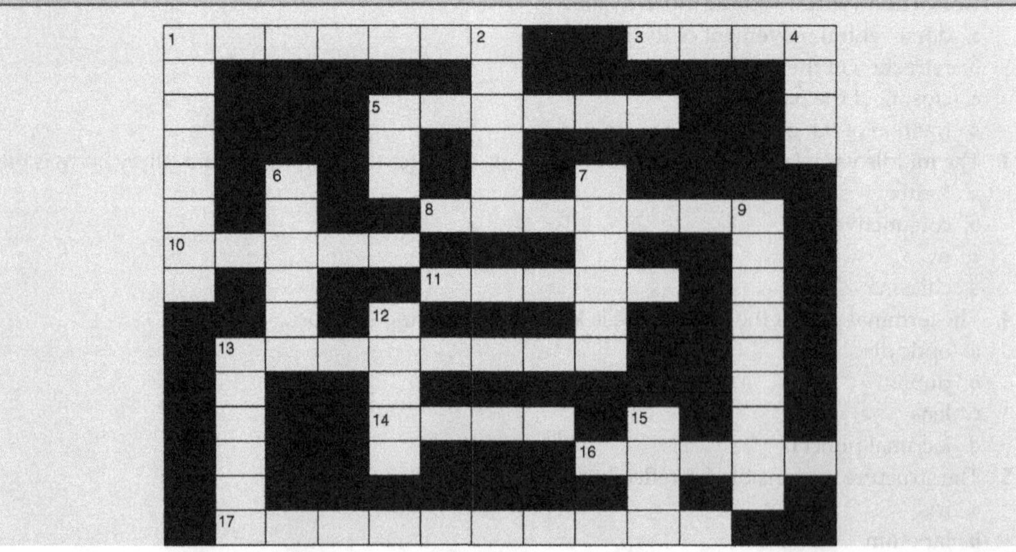

Exercise 5.20

Across	Down
1. This humour is found in the anterior and posterior chambers	1. This chamber is between the cornea and the iris.
3. This film is mostly lacrimal fluid.	2. The 'white' of the eye.
5. Pupils do this in poor light.	4. The photoreceptors associated with black and white vision.
8. The shiny inner layer of the choroids.	5. The species with eyelashes.
10. Cranial nerve II.	6. The nervous inner layer of the globe.
11. The hole in the centre of the iris.	7. The inner canthus.
13. A gland that produces tears.	9. The glands in the eyelid producing a fatty secretion.
14. The muscular pigmented part of the eye.	12. The eye socket.
16. This point is what the animal is looking at.	13. The junction of the sclera and cornea.
17. These ligaments hold the lens in place.	15. The number of lacrimal punctae.

Multiple choice questions – the ear

Exercise 5.21

1. The auricular cartilage:
   a. makes up the pinna
   b. surrounds the auditory canal
   c. separates the outer and middle ear
   d. is the organ of balance.
2. Ceruminous glands are modified:
   a. sudoriferous glands
   b. sebaceous glands
   c. mucous glands
   d. mammary glands.
3. The auditory ossicle attached to the vestibular window is the:
   a. malleus
   b. incus
   c. stapes
   d. annular cartilage.
4. The auditory tube opens out into the:
   a. oropharynx
   b. inner ear
   c. outer ear
   d. nasopharynx.
5. The bony labyrinth is:
   a. plasma filled
   b. endolymph filled
   c. air filled
   d. perilymph filled.

6. The endolymphatic sac is found in the:
   a. epidural space
   b. tympanic bulla
   c. subarachnoid space
   d. external acoustic meatus.

Tip: *Why not get together with fellow students and write some more questions for each other?*

Activity

Exercise 5.22 Below is a diagram of the ear. From the selection, add the correct labels

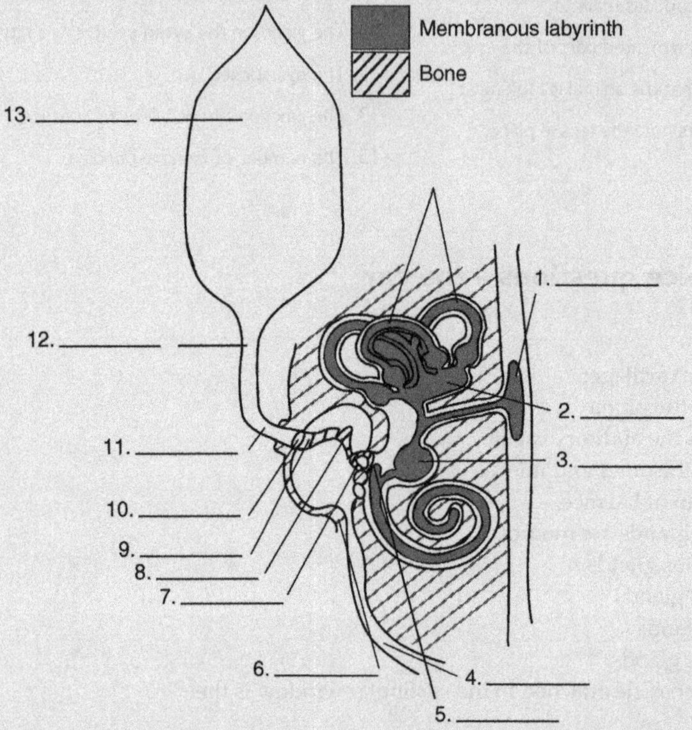

Stapes	Vertical canal	Tympanic bulla	Saccule	
Pinna	Utricle	Horizontal canal	Incus	Tympanic membrane
Malleus	Vestibular window	Endolymphatic sac	Auditory Tube	

Figure 5.9 Diagram of the ear.
(Reproduced with kind permission from Lane & Cooper 1999.)

CHAPTER 6

The endocrine system

LEARNING Objectives

This chapter will help you to revise the following:

- facts and functions of the endocrine system
- the pituitary gland
- the thyroid gland
- the parathyroid glands
- the adrenal glands
- the pancreas
- the gonads
- other endocrine tissues.

There is a general revision section at the end of the chapter.

Facts and functions of the endocrine system

1. The endocrine system consists of the following components:
   a. endocrine glands, made from epithelial tissue and producing secretions called hormones
   b. other endocrine tissue in various organs of the body also secreting hormones
   c. the bloodstream, which acts as a transport system for the hormones to reach their sites of action or target organs.
2. Hormones are categorized into two main groups, according to their chemical composition:
   a. steroid hormones
   b. protein hormones.
3. The endocrine system and hormones have a major regulatory function in the body. Their effects can be split into four main groups:
   a. metabolic (controlling the rate and balance of chemical reactions)
   b. kinetic (allowing the movement of substances around the body)
   c. behavioural (controlling behaviour)
   d. morphogenetic (changing the appearance and structure of tissues).
4. Many hormones fall into more than one of the above categories.
5. Hormone secretion has a resting (basal) level that alters in response to various stimuli:
   a. nervous system
   b. other hormones
   c. extracellular environment.
6. This system of altering hormone production in response to information received is known as a *feedback loop*.
7. If hormone production drops in response to information received, the system is called a *negative* feedback loop; this is very common in the animal body and serves to keep hormone production in check.
8. If hormone production increases in response to information received, the system is called a *positive* feedback loop; this is less common in the animal body but is found when sudden, large amounts of hormone are required, e.g. to trigger ovulation.

The pituitary gland

Key Points:

1. The pituitary gland is situated at the base of the brain, connected to the hypothalamus. It is sometimes referred to as the 'master gland'.

2. The pituitary gland is separated into two parts:
   a. the anterior pituitary, or adenohypophysis, which secretes six hormones:
      i. FSH (follicle-stimulating hormone), which stimulates the ovarian follicles in the female and spermatogenesis in the male
      ii. ACTH (adrenocorticotrophic hormone), which stimulates the adrenal cortex
      iii. somatotrophin (a growth hormone), which controls growth rate, mainly of bone tissue
      iv. TSH (thyroid-stimulating hormone or thyrotrophin), which regulates the release of the thyroid hormones
      v. LH (luteinizing hormone), which acts on the ovary to stimulate ovulation. In the male, the hormone is sometimes called ICSH (interstitial cell-stimulating hormone), which stimulates testosterone production
      vi. prolactin; this hormone stimulates mammary development and milk production in late pregnancy.
   b. The posterior pituitary, or neurohypophysis, is actually a storage area for two hormones secreted by the hypothalamus:
      i. ADH (antidiuretic hormone or vasopressin), which targets the renal tubules to increase the reabsorption of water and therefore concentrate the urine
      ii. oxytocin; this causes the smooth muscle in the uterine wall to contract during parturition. It also acts on the mammary ducts to allow milk letdown.

Activity

Exercise 6.1 Draw a chart depicting the hormones of the pituitary gland, their sites of action and their functions.

Mnemonic

To remember the hormones of the anterior pituitary gland.

Fast lip

FSH
ACTH
Somatotrophin
TSH
LH/ICSH
Prolactin

The thyroid gland

Key Points:

1. The thyroid gland is a paired gland with one lobe on either side of the proximal trachea, situated laterally.
2. The thyroid gland produces three hormones:
   a. thyroxin or T4
   b. tri-iodothyronine or T3
   c. thyrocalcitonin or calcitonin.
3. T4 and T3 have similar functions, which involve regulating metabolism.
4. Thyrocalcitonin decreases calcium uptake from the bones, so is produced in response to a high blood calcium level.

Look it up

Exercise 6.2 Hyperthyroidism is a common condition in cats, and hypothyroidism is sometimes seen in dogs. In the table below, list the symptoms seen with these conditions. This will help you to understand the functions of the thyroid gland.

Symptoms	Hyperthyroidism	Hypothyroidism
Heart rate	(1)	(2)
Respiratory rate	(3)	(4)
Skin condition	(5)	(6)
Coat condition	(7)	(8)
Bodyweight	(9)	(10)
General demeanour	(11)	(12)

The parathyroid glands

Key Points:

1. The parathyroid glands are four tiny structures.
2. Each lobe of the thyroid gland has two parathyroid glands—one on its surface and one deep within its centre.
3. The parathyroid glands produce PTH (parathyroid hormone or parathormone).
4. PTH increases calcium uptake from the bones in response to a low blood calcium level, i.e. it has the opposite function to thyrocalcitonin.

The adrenal glands

Key Points:

1. There are two adrenal glands, one on the craniomedial surface of each kidney.
2. Each adrenal gland comprises an outer cortex and inner medulla.
3. The adrenal cortex produces the following:
   a. glucocorticoids (cortisol and corticosterone), which carry out a number of functions including increasing blood glucose levels by gluconeogenesis (producing glucose from a number of other metabolites such as amino acids), mobilization of fat stores and stimulation of appetite. Levels of glucocorticoid increase if the animal is stressed. Very high levels have an anti-inflammatory effect on the body
   b. mineralocorticoids (aldosterone is the main mineralocorticoid), which regulate the levels of ions in the body, especially sodium and potassium.
4. The adrenal medulla produces adrenaline and noradrenaline (also called epinephrine and norepinephrine, respectively); these are the 'fight or flight' hormones and prepare the body for an emergency. Their actions include increasing heart and respiratory rates, increasing blood glucose and dilating arteries.
5. The adrenal glands also produce the sex hormones at a low level.

Activity

Exercise 6.3 Draw a chart depicting the hormones of the adrenal glands, their sites of action and their functions.

The Pancreas

Key Points:

1. The pancreas is a V-shaped organ situated alongside the stomach and duodenum.
2. The pancreas is a *mixed gland*, meaning it has both endocrine and exocrine functions.
3. The exocrine part of the pancreas produces pancreatic juice, used for digestion (see Ch. 9, 'The Digestive System', for more information).
4. The endocrine parts of the pancreas are known as the Islets of Langerhans. The Islets produce three hormones:
   a. glucagon, produced by the alpha cells in response to low blood glucose levels, turns glycogen in the liver into glucose, which is then released into the bloodstream
   b. insulin, produced by the beta cells in response to a high blood glucose level, allows the uptake of glucose into cells from the bloodstream and prevents breakdown of glycogen and gluconeogenesis
   c. somatostatin, produced by the delta cells, moderates the action of both glucagon and insulin.

Activity

Exercise 6.4 Diabetes mellitus is a common condition in dogs, caused by little or no production of insulin or insensitivity to insulin. In the table below, list the symptoms seen with this condition along with their causes. This will help you to understand the function of insulin.

Parameter	Symptom	Reason
Appetite	(1)	(2)
Bodyweight	(3)	(4)
Blood	(5)	(6)
Urine	(7)	(8)
Thirst	(9)	(10)

The gonads

Key Points:

1. The gonads, i.e. the ovaries in the female and the testicles in the male, are discussed in more detail in Ch. 11 ('The Reproductive System').
2. The ovaries produce the following hormones:
   a. oestradiol, an oestrogen produced by cells in the ovarian wall that causes the signs of oestrus and prepares the genital tract for mating
   b. progesterone (produced by the corpus luteum); its function is to maintain pregnancy
   c. relaxin (also produced by the corpus luteum in late pregnancy), causes relaxation of ligaments in preparation for parturition.

3. The testicles produce the following hormones:
   a. testosterone, an androgen produced by the Leydig cells. Its function is to promote spermatogenesis and to develop and maintain secondary male characteristics, e.g. scent marking, territoriality and sex drive
   b. oestrogen, produced by the Sertoli cells. It is thought to act as a 'balance' to testosterone.

Activity

Exercise 6.5 Draw a chart depicting the hormones of the gonads, their sites of action and their functions.

Mnemonic

To remember the function of the female sex hormones.
Oestrogen: **O** is for **o**estrus symptoms
Progesterone: **P** is for **p**regnancy maintenance

Other endocrine tissues

Key Points:

There are several other areas of the body that produce hormones, for example:
1. The stomach wall; produces gastrin, a hormone that stimulates the production of hydrochloric acid.
2. The small intestine; produces secretin, a hormone that stimulates the production of digestive juices.
3. The placenta; produces chorionic gonadotrophin, a hormone that maintains the corpus luteum throughout pregnancy.

General revision

Multiple choice questions

Exercise 6.6

1. A negative feedback loop causes:
   a. increased production of a hormone
   b. a different hormone to be produced
   c. decreased production of a hormone
   d. hormone production to remain the same.
2. ACTH stands for:
   a. adrenocorticotrophic hormone
   b. adrenocorticothyroid hormone
   c. aminocorticothyroid hormone
   d. aminocorticotrophic hormone.
3. Gluconeogenesis occurs in response to:
   a. mineralocorticoid production
   b. insulin production

c. glucocorticoid production
d. PTH production.

4. TSH is produced by the:
   a. thyroid gland
   b. anterior pituitary gland
   c. parathyroid gland
   d. posterior pituitary.
5. Adrenaline is also known as:
   a. epinephrine
   b. neurohypophysis
   c. calcitonin
   d. oestradiol.
6. Aldosterone is a:
   a. androgen
   b. oestrogen
   c. glucocorticoid
   d. mineralocorticoid.
7. Pregnancy is maintained by:
   a. oestradiol
   b. relaxin
   c. progesterone
   d. prolactin.
8. The corpus luteum produces:
   a. oestradiol
   b. relaxin
   c. prolactin
   d. testosterone.
9. The pancreas produces:
   a. glucocorticoid
   b. glucagon
   c. ACTH
   d. ADH.
10. The target organ for ADH is the:
    a. liver
    b. renal tubules
    c. ovary
    d. thyroid gland.
11. Cortisol causes:
    a. an increase in blood glucose
    b. an increase in water reabsorption
    c. a decrease in blood glucose
    d. a decrease in heart rate.
12. The target organ for somatotrophin is mainly the:
    a. heart
    b. kidney
    c. bones
    d. liver.

13. Secondary male characteristics are caused by:
    a. FSH
    b. oestrogen
    c. TSH
    d. testosterone.
14. PTH causes:
    a. an increase in blood calcium levels
    b. an increase in blood glucose levels
    c. a decrease in blood calcium levels
    d. a decrease in blood glucose levels.
15. Insulin causes:
    a. an increase in blood calcium levels
    b. an increase in blood glucose levels
    c. a decrease in blood calcium levels
    d. a decrease in blood glucose levels.
16. ICSH is another term for:
    a. ACTH
    b. TSH
    c. ADH
    d. LH.
17. Noradrenaline is produced in the:
    a. adrenal cortex
    b. adrenal medulla
    c. pancreas
    d. placenta.
18. Secretin is produced by the:
    a. stomach
    b. liver
    c. small intestine
    d. large intestine.
19. Oxytocin causes:
    a. uterine smooth muscle contraction
    b. relaxation of ligaments prior to parturition
    c. mammary development
    d. maintenance of pregnancy.
20. Aldosterone:
    a. maintains pregnancy
    b. maintains ion balance
    c. moderates the adrenal cortex
    d. moderates the action of insulin.

Tip: *Why not get together with fellow students and write some more questions for each other?*

Activity

Design a poster on A3 paper depicting the position of the endocrine glands in the dog. Include with each label a list of the hormones produced by that endocrine gland. Use large labels and bold colours. When it is complete, stick it where you will regularly read it. Why not on a kitchen cupboard?

Study

Exercise 6.7 Once you have found all the hormones listed below in the wordsearch grid, write down their target organs and functions.

Hormone	Target organ	Function
Gastrin		
Prolactin		
Thyroxin		
Vasopressin		
Relaxin		
Oxytocin		
Glucagon		
Aldosterone		

V	A	S	O	P	R	E	S	S	I	N
A	L	G	I	O	L	U	I	G	O	S
S	D	T	L	X	E	C	N	A	X	T
N	O	S	H	U	N	A	O	S	Y	E
I	S	X	T	Y	C	G	T	X	T	R
T	T	H	A	T	R	A	I	T	O	X
C	E	Y	L	O	O	O	G	A	C	T
A	R	I	O	C	Y	N	X	O	I	H
L	O	N	G	A	S	T	R	I	N	R
O	N	R	E	L	A	X	I	N	N	Y
R	E	S	R	I	H	C	C	A	O	O
P	A	O	P	N	T	A	L	L	D	S

Activity

Exercise 6.8 True or false? If the statement is false, write the corrected statement in the relevant space.

Statement	True or false
The anterior pituitary gland is also called the neurohypophysis	(1)
The thyroid gland is a paired structure	(2)
Parathormone causes an increase in blood calcium levels	(3)
The adrenal cortex produces adrenaline	(4)
The Islets of Langerhans produce pancreatic juice	(5)

Statement	True or false
Testosterone is produced by the Leydig cells	(6)
Oestrogen is produced by the corpus luteum	(7)
The placenta produces chorionic gonadotrophin	(8)

Activity

Prepare a ten-minute presentation entitled 'The hormones of the adrenal cortex'. Your audience could be family, friends or fellow students. When you have finished, invite questions from the floor!

CHAPTER 7

The heart and blood vascular system, and lymphatic and immune systems

LEARNING Objectives

This chapter will help you to revise the following:

- facts and functions of the heart
- the anatomy of the heart
- the flow of blood through the heart
- contraction of the heart
- the cardiac cycle and blood pressure
- facts about blood
- blood plasma and its constituents
- erythrocytes
- leucocytes
- thrombocytes and the clotting mechanism
- the structure of blood vessels
- the circulation
- the major blood vessels
- facts and functions of the lymphatic system
- lymph
- lymph vessels
- lymph nodes
- other areas of lymphatic tissue
- facts and functions of the immune system
- humoral immunity
- cellular immunity
- phagocytosis.

There is a general revision section at the end of the chapter.

THE HEART AND BLOOD VASCULAR SYSTEM

Facts and functions of the heart

1. The function of the heart is to pump blood around the body (systemic circulation) and to the lungs to be oxygenated (pulmonary circulation).
2. The heart is found in the ventral thoracic cavity within the mediastinum. It lies slightly to the left on the sagittal plane, parallel with rib pairs 3 to 6.
3. The major vessels supplying blood to the heart are found at its base, which is more dorsocranial than the opposite end (the apex).
4. The prefix denoting the heart is *cardio–*.

Activity

Draw the correct position of the heart on the following diagrams.

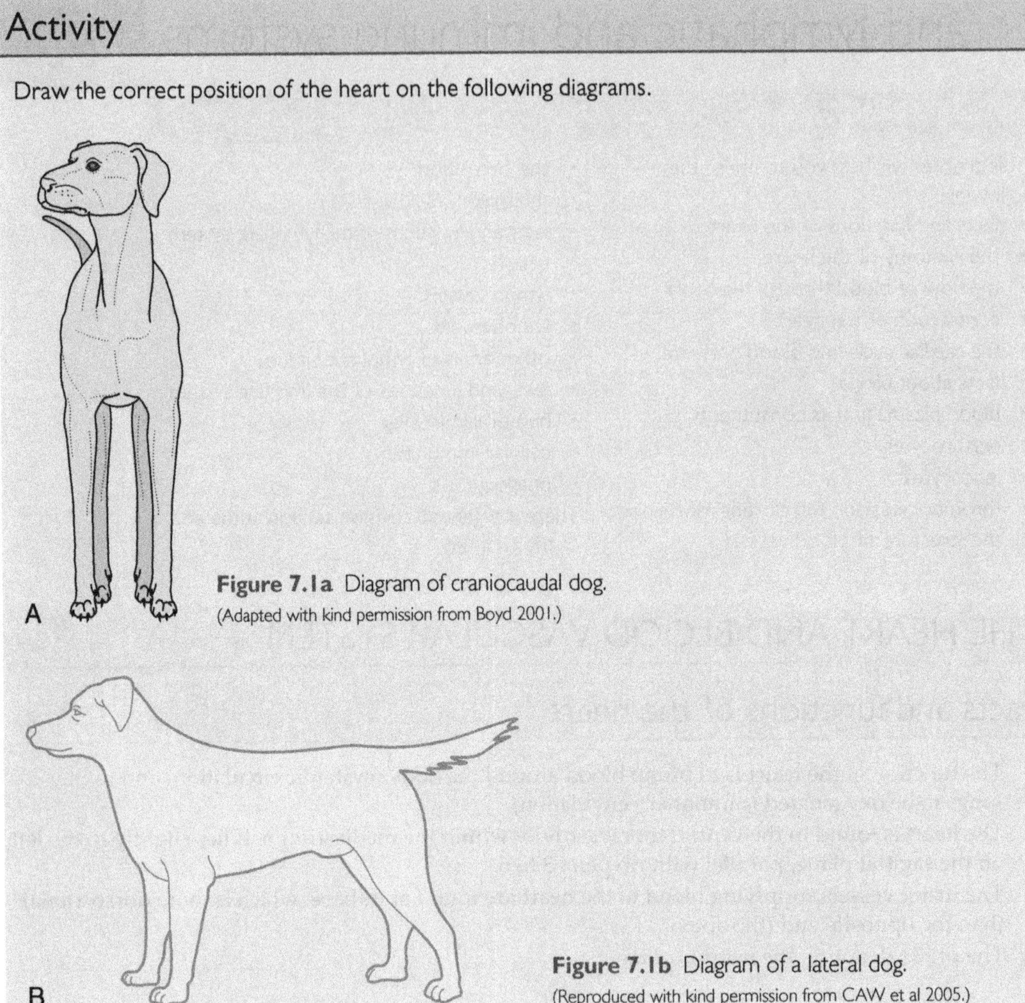

Figure 7.1a Diagram of craniocaudal dog.
(Adapted with kind permission from Boyd 2001.)

Figure 7.1b Diagram of a lateral dog.
(Reproduced with kind permission from CAW et al 2005.)

The anatomy of the heart

Key Points:

1. The heart is a roughly cone-shaped structure made up largely of muscle tissue (myocardium).
2. A serous sac (the pericardium) surrounds the heart. At the heart's base, the pericardium is fused to the myocardium to form the epicardium.
3. There are four chambers inside the heart—two on the right and two on the left. The two sides are separated by the cardiac septum.
4. The upper two chambers are the right and left atria (singular, atrium).
5. The lower two chambers are the right and left ventricles.
6. Valves and attached chordae tendinae arise from papillary muscles, which project from the inner walls of the ventricles.

Activity

Exercise 7.1 Below is a diagram of a heart. From the selection, add the correct labels.

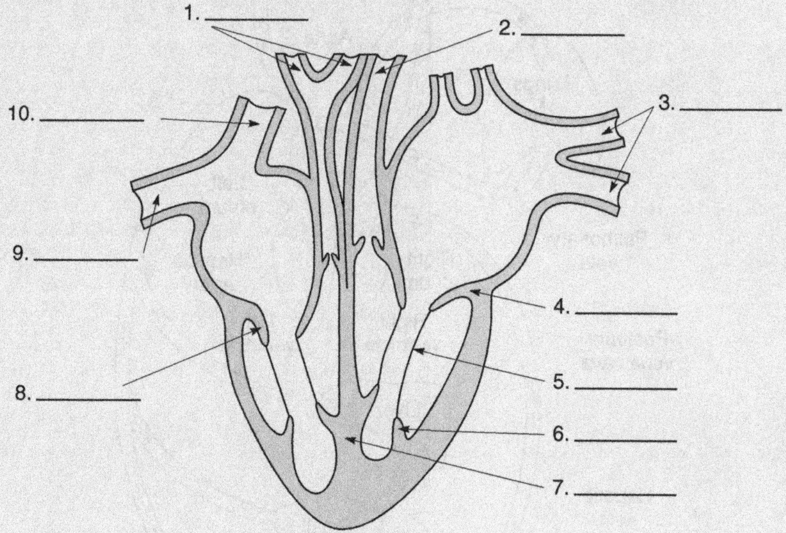

Anterior vena cava	Chorda tendina	Aorta	Right atrioventricular valve
Pulmonary arteries	Papillary muscle	Interventricular septum	Pulmonary veins
Posterior vena cava	Left atrioventricular valve		

Figure 7.2 Cross-section through a heart to show the structure.
(Reproduced with permission from Bowden & Masters 2001.)

The flow of blood through the heart

Key Points:

1. Blood follows a specific route through the heart and only flows in one direction.
2. The blood entering the chambers does not supply the myocardium; this is served by the coronary arteries.
3. Valves prevent the backflow of blood.
4. Blood from the right and left sides of the heart does not mix as blood in the right side is deoxygenated and blood in the left side is oxygenated.

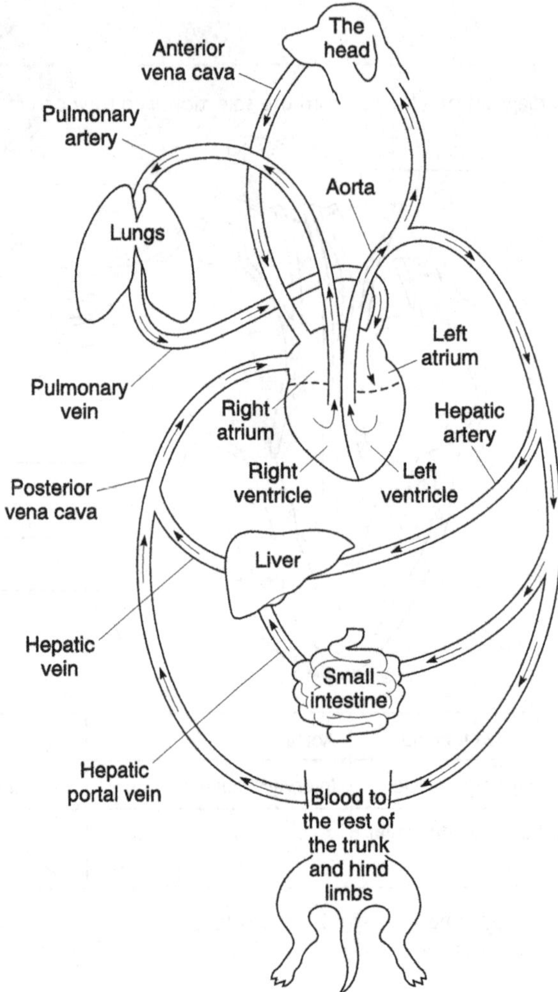

Figure 7.3 Schematic diagram of the heart with circulations showing the direction of blood flow.
(Reproduced with permission from Bowden & Masters 2001.)

List the structures

Exercise 7.2 From the selection of structures below, construct a flowchart to show the route an erythrocyte would take through the heart, beginning with the vena cava.

Vena cava	Pulmonary artery	Right ventricle
Right atrioventricular valve	Aorta	Around the body to distribute oxygen
Lungs to be oxygenated	Left atrioventricular valve	Pulmonary vein
Pulmonary semilunar valve	Right atrium	Aortic semilunar valve
Left atrium	Left ventricle	

Contraction of the heart

Key Points:

1. The 'pacemaker' of the heart stimulates contraction.
2. The rate of contraction is decided by a number of factors including:
   a. stimulation of the autonomic nervous system
   b. the physical condition of the animal and presence of disease
   c. stretch receptors in the heart, which respond to a change in blood pressure.

Table 7.1 Normal heart rates in dogs and cats. (Adapted, with permission, from Lane & Cooper 1999.)

	Dog	Cat
Pulse (beats per minute)	60–180 (depending on size of breed)	110–180

Fill in the gaps

Exercise 7.3 Complete the paragraph on the contraction of the heart by filling in the gaps using the correct words from the selection below.

- systole
- diastole
- atria
- Purkinje
- fibrillation
- bundle
- pacemaker
- myocardium

There are three specialized areas in the (1)__________, which are linked by a conduction system made of (2)__________ tissue:

- sinuatrial node, found in the wall of the right atrium and known as the (3)__________
- atrioventricular node and atrioventricular (4)__________, found between the atrium and ventricles.

Impulses move from the sinuatrial node across the (5)__________ to cause their contraction. The impulses then reach the atrioventricular node and bundle, causing ventricular contraction. Contraction of heart muscle is known as (6)__________ and relaxation of heart muscle is known as (7)__________. A healthy heart will be synchronized so that during atrial contraction there is ventricular relaxation and vice versa. Certain diseases sometimes cause problems with this conduction system so that the muscle fibres within a certain area of the heart are not contracting together; this is known as (8)__________.

The cardiac cycle and blood pressure

Key Points:

1. The cardiac cycle is one complete heartbeat. All the processes that occur during a heartbeat are part of the cardiac cycle.
2. The two distinct sounds (usually described as 'lub-dub') are mainly caused by the closing of the valves:
   a. 'lub' is the atrioventricular valves closing during ventricular systole
   b. 'dub' is the semilunar valves closing during ventricular diastole.
3. Blood pressure is the pressure in the blood vessels. It is usually arterial blood pressure that is measured.

4. Blood pressure is at its highest during ventricular systole and at its lowest during ventricular diastole. Normally both pressures are measured and expressed in units of millimetres of mercury (mmHg) as depicted below:

$$\frac{\text{Ventricular systolic pressure (mmHg)}}{\text{Ventricular diastolic pressure (mmHg)}}$$

5. Normal canine and feline blood pressure is approximately 180/100, although this depends on the site and method used to take the measurement.
6. Blood pressure is regulated by the autonomic nervous system and the endocrine system.

The sequence of events during the cardiac cycle

The flowchart below shows the sequence of events that occur during the cardiac cycle.

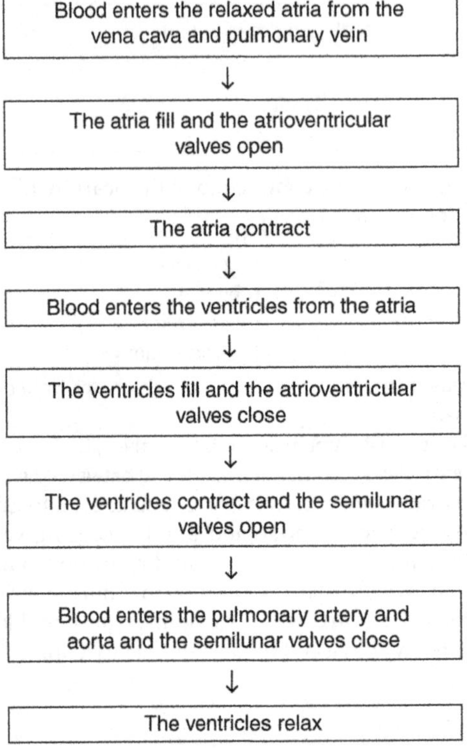

Facts about blood

1. Blood is classed as a connective tissue.
2. Blood is red due to the haemoglobin content of erythrocytes.
3. Blood makes up 5 to 10% of bodyweight.
4. The pH of blood is approximately 7.4.
5. The prefix denoting blood is *haem–*.
6. The functions of blood are:
   a. transportation of various substances around the body including:
      i. oxygen and carbon dioxide
      ii. nutrients

   iii. waste products
   iv. hormones and enzymes
   v. distribution of heat from the liver and muscles.
b. body defence:
   i. immunoglobulins (or antibodies) are proteins produced by certain leucocytes in response to antigens
   ii. other leucocytes present in the bloodstream engulf foreign matter by phagocytosis
   iii. the clotting mechanism prevents blood loss if damage to circulation occurs.
c. fluid balance and pH maintenance:
   i. replenishment of interstitial fluid
   ii. the plasma protein albumin maintains blood osmotic pressure
   iii. the salt compounds in blood act as buffers to maintain the correct acid–base balance of body fluid.

Fill in the gaps

Exercise 7.4 Complete the paragraph below, on the functions of blood, by filling in the gaps using the correct words from the selection below.

- transport
- haemoglobin
- defence
- albumin
- hormones
- 7.4
- heat
- clotting
- 5–10
- oxygen

Blood makes up (1)__________% of bodyweight and is pH (2)__________. It is red in colour due to the (3)__________ content of erythrocytes. The higher the degree of (4)__________ saturation of haemoglobin, the brighter the colour. One of the main functions of blood is to (5)__________ substances around the body, including oxygen, carbon dioxide, nutrients and waste products. Blood is also the transport medium for the secretions of endocrine glands (6)(__________) and distributes (7)__________ from the muscles and liver. The blood also contains leucocytes, which are involved in body (8)__________. If the vascular system is damaged in any way, it will be repaired by the (9)__________ mechanism. Blood osmotic pressure is maintained mainly by the plasma protein (10)__________.

Activity

Exercise 7.5 Examine the mucous membranes of several dogs and cats. Make a note of the colour and capillary refill time. Consider why these parameters vary and which conditions could cause abnormal results. Complete the chart below:

Mucous membrane colour	Possible cause
Pale or white	(1)
Blue-grey (cyanotic)	(2)
Yellow tinged	(3)
Brick red	(4)
Chocolate brown	(5)

Blood plasma

Key Points:

1. Plasma is the liquid component of blood in which the blood cells are suspended.
2. Plasma comprises water, salt compounds (sodium, potassium, etc.) and proteins among other substances.
3. Normal plasma is clear and straw coloured in the dog and cat.
4. Serum is plasma without the presence of clotting factors.

Activity

Exercise 7.6 The following components of plasma are hidden in the wordsearch grid below. How many can you find?

- Albumin
- Clotting factors
- Immunoglobulins
- Salts
- Leucocytes
- Erythrocytes
- Water
- Hormones
- Thrombocytes
- Urea
- Nutrients

E	L	E	Y	A	U	T	F	L	B	W	T	B	U	I
R	E	R	R	H	N	O	A	A	U	R	A	R	T	M
T	U	Y	C	Y	U	L	L	S	S	O	E	T	H	M
H	C	T	S	K	T	C	H	E	A	H	R	E	A	U
C	O	H	E	E	R	H	A	A	L	B	U	M	I	N
U	C	M	T	L	I	E	R	T	T	U	H	I	W	O
R	Y	B	Y	H	E	U	T	O	S	Q	R	M	A	G
Q	T	M	C	T	N	B	C	Y	C	W	O	O	T	L
U	E	I	O	G	T	R	L	C	O	Y	M	R	E	O
L	S	N	B	W	S	U	M	I	T	U	T	H	R	B
U	E	I	M	R	O	B	C	M	T	B	B	E	E	U
R	B	H	O	R	M	O	N	E	S	O	O	T	S	L
S	U	M	R	J	T	L	T	S	F	L	N	Y	T	I
T	I	M	H	F	H	A	O	R	A	G	E	R	P	N
C	L	O	T	T	I	N	G	F	A	C	T	O	R	S

Erythrocytes

Key points:

1. An erythrocyte is a mature red blood cell. (See Ch. 1, 'Body Composition and Cells', for general revision of cells).
2. The smallest and most numerous blood cell, erythrocytes are 7 micrometres (μm) in diameter and there are approximately 7,000,000 per microlitre (μL) of blood.

3. Erythrocytes are bilaterally concave in shape and, when mature, lack a nucleus.
4. Oxygen combines with the haemoglobin in the erythrocytes to form oxyhaemoglobin. This is how oxygen is transported around the body.

Erythrocyte production

Erythrocyte production is called *erythropoiesis* and in the fetus it occurs in the liver, spleen and bone marrow. After birth it occurs almost exclusively in the bone marrow (myeloid tissue).

Activity

Exercise 7.7 Put the following points in the correct order to construct a chart to show the sequence of events during erythrocyte production.

(1) More erythrocytes enter the bloodstream, so more haemoglobin is present.	(2) Erythropoietin factor converts a plasma protein into erythropoietin, which is needed for erythrocyte production.
(3) Erythropoietin factor is released from the kidneys in response to poor oxygen supply.	(4) The oxygen deficit is reduced.
(5) Erythropoietin causes increased erythrocyte production in the myeloid tissue.	(6) Oxygen levels in the body tissues drop.
(7) Erythrocytes break down at the ends of their lives.	

Erythrocyte development

1. *Erythroblasts* develop into *normoblasts* as they take up haemoglobin.
2. Normoblasts develop into *reticulocytes* as the nucleus is broken down.
3. Reticulocytes become *erythrocytes* as the nucleus disappears completely; at this stage they are released into the bloodstream.
4. It is not unusual to find a small number of reticulocytes in the bloodstream; an increased amount suggests *regenerative anaemia*.
5. The spleen is a storage site for erythrocytes.
6. Erythrocytes have a life-span of approximately 110 days, after which time they are broken down. Some components of the erythrocyte, e.g. the iron, are recycled but some are excreted, e.g. bilirubin is a product of haemoglobin breakdown which is excreted in the urine and faeces.

Leucocytes

Key Points:

1. A leucocyte is a white blood cell. (See Ch. 1, 'Body Composition and Cells', for general revision of cells).
2. Leucocytes are larger and less numerous than erythrocytes.
3. There are five main types of leucocyte, all of which play a part in the body's defences.
4. All leucocytes are produced in the myeloid tissue, although one type, lymphocytes, differentiate and develop in the lymphoid tissue.

Types of leucocyte

The following diagram shows the different types of leucocyte.

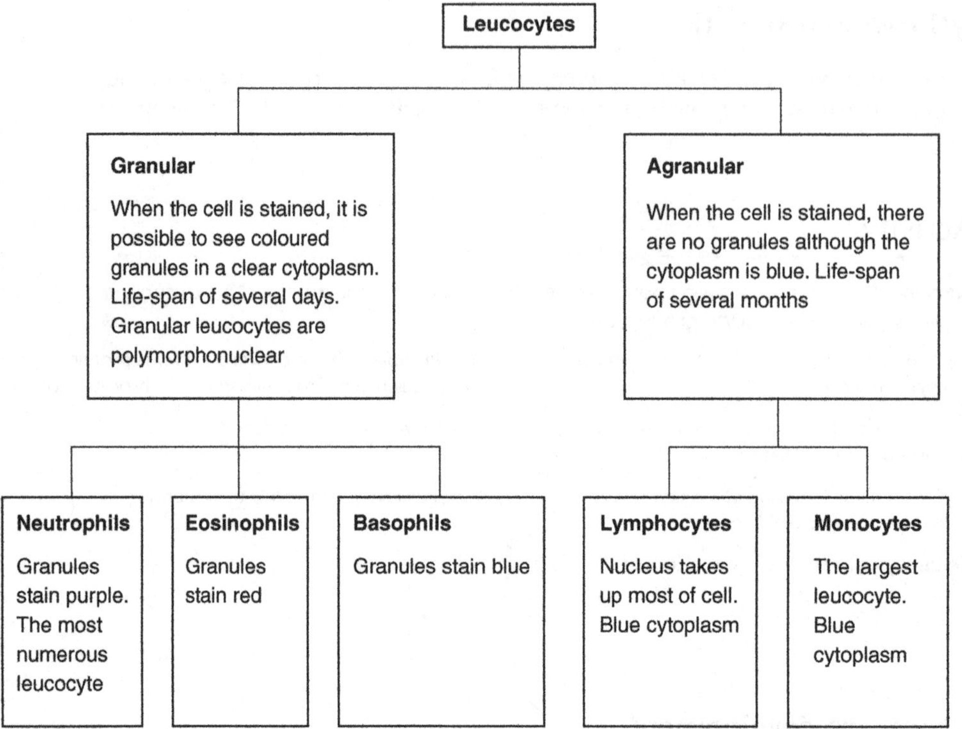

Figure 7.4 Types of leucocyte.

Link the words

Exercise 7.8 Match the description in the left-hand column to the correct definition in the right-hand column by drawing a line to link them.

(1)There are two main types: T-cells and B-cells. T-cells destroy diseased cells and B-cells produce antibodies	(2)Neutrophil
(3)Phagocytic cell, which is also found in other body tissues, where it is called a macrophage	(4)Eosinophil
(5)Destroys foreign matter such as bacteria by phagocytosis. Present in large numbers in pus	(6)Basophil
(7)Phagocytic cell which increases in number during parasitic or allergic disease	(8)Lymphocyte
(9)Produces histamine and is present in increased numbers during allergic or parasitic disease	(10)Monocyte

Activity

Design a poster on A3 paper depicting the different types of leucocyte. Use large labels and bold colours. When it is complete, stick it where you will regularly read it. Why not on a kitchen cupboard?

Table 7.2 The normal ranges of total and differential leucocytes. (Adapted with permission from Lane & Cooper 1999.)

Parameter	Units	Canine	Feline	Equine	Thoroughbred	Bovine	Ovine
WBCs	10^9/l	6–15	4–15	6–12	7–14	3.5–10	4–10
Lymphocytes	10^9/l	1–4.8	1.5–6.5	1–6	1.7–9.8	1–4.6	2.6–7.2
	%	12–30	25–33	15–50	25–70	40–60	65–72
Mature neutrophils	10^9/l	3.6–10.5	2.5–12.5	2.1–9	2.1–9	0.7–4.9	0.7–3.2
	%	60–70	45–75	35–75	30–65	21–49	18–32
Band neutrophils	10^9/l	0–0.3	0–0.45	0–0.24	0–0.28	0–0.2	0–0.1
	%	0–2	0–3	0–2	0–2	0–2	0–1
Eosinophils	10^9/l	0.1–1.5	0.1–1.8	0.1–1.4	0–1.5	0–1.6	0–10.
	%	2–10	4–12	2–12	1–11	0–16	0–10
Monocytes	10^9/l	0.18–1.5	0–0.6	0.12–1.2	0–1	0–1	0–1
	%	3–10	0–4	2–10	0.5–7.0	2–10	0–10
Basophils	10^9/l	0	0	0–0.3	0–0.4	0	0–0.2
	%	rare	rare	0–3	0–3	rare	0–2
Platelets	10^9/l	200–500	200–600	90–500	100–300	200–300	200–700

Source: Bloxham Laboratories Ltd, Teignmouth, Devon

Thrombocytes and the clotting mechanism

Key Points:

1. Thrombocytes are also known as platelets.
2. Thrombocytes are not true cells but fragments of large cells in the myeloid tissue known as *megakaryocytes*.
3. Thrombocytes play an important part in blood clotting, along with substances known as clotting factors (special proteins, which are mostly produced in the liver).
4 Many clotting factors depend on vitamin K for their formation.
5. Heparin, a natural anticoagulant, prevents clotting in areas where it is not wanted.

The clotting mechanism or 'coagulation cascade'

Activity

Exercise 7.9 Place the following sequence of events in the order in which they occur.

(1)The normal blood clotting time of dogs and cats is 2.5 to 5 minutes.	(2)Thrombin acts on another clotting factor, fibrinogen, to produce fibrin.
(3)Damage to the blood vessel wall.	(4)Thrombocytes stick to the wound site and produce the enzyme thromboplastin.
(5)Fibrin sticks to thrombocytes to form a mesh over the wound; this is a clot.	(6)Thromboplastin combines with calcium in the blood to turn the clotting factor prothrombin into the enzyme thrombin.

The structure of blood vessels

Key Points:

1. There are three main types of blood vessel:
   a. arteries
   b. veins
   c. capillaries.
2. These blood vessels link to form a network throughout the entire body through which blood flows.

Activity

Exercise 7.10 Below are diagrams of the different blood vessels. On each diagram, add the correct labels.

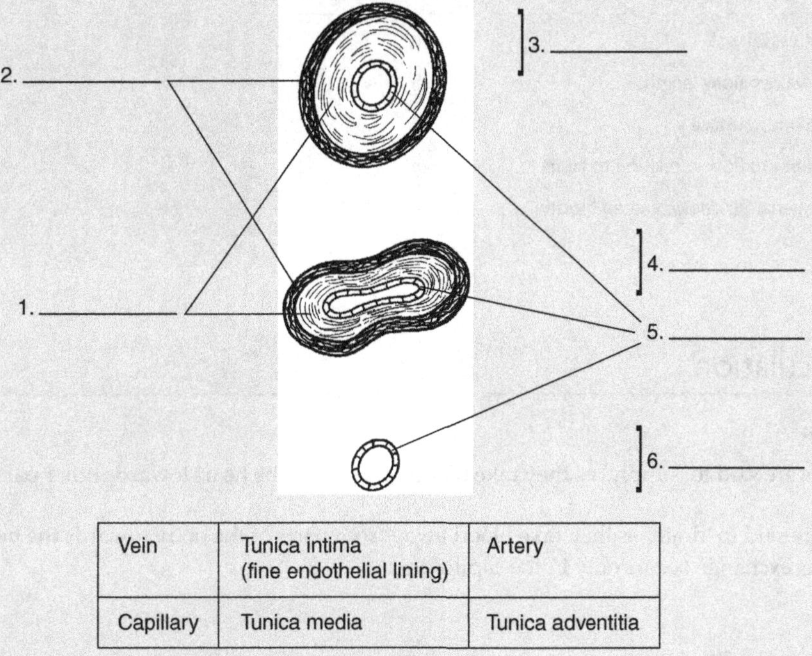

Vein	Tunica intima (fine endothelial lining)	Artery
Capillary	Tunica media	Tunica adventitia

Figure 7.5 The structures of an artery, vein and a capillary (not to scale).
(Adapted with permission from Lane & Cooper 1999.)

Link the words

Exercise 7.11 Match the description in the left-hand column to the correct definition in the right-hand column by drawing a line to link them.

(1)A small vein within the organ it is draining	(2)Artery
(3)A fine vessel through whose walls gaseous exchange takes place	(4)Vein
(5)Thick-walled vessel carrying blood away from the heart	(6)Capillary
(7)A small branching type of artery found only in the brain, heart and kidney	(8)Arteriole
(9)Thin-walled vessel carrying blood to the heart	(10)Venule
(11)A small artery within the organ it is supplying	(12)End artery

Activity

Exercise 7.12 Complete the chart below to depict the differences between arteries and veins.

Feature	Arteries	Veins
Thickness of vessel wall	(1)	(2)
Presence of valves along length	(3)	(4)
Proximity to body surface	(5)	(6)
Direction of blood flow in relation to heart	(7)	(8)
Carrying oxygenated/deoxygenated blood	(9)	(10)

The circulation

Key Points:

1. Arteries are said to 'supply' as they take blood away from the heart towards other parts of the body.
2. Veins are said to 'drain' as they take blood away from parts of the body towards the heart.
3. Gaseous exchange occurs only in the capillaries.

Categories of circulation

Different types of circulation are sometimes described:

1. *The pulmonary circulation*, which supplies blood to the lungs where it is oxygenated and returns it back to the heart.
2. *The systemic circulation*, which supplies blood to the rest of the body and returns it back to the heart.
3. *Fetal circulation*, which refers to the circulation in the unborn animal. There are several differences between this and the animal after birth. Describe these differences in the box below.

(Continued)

4. *Portal circulation*, which is a vein (or group of veins) where both ends terminate in a capillary bed. A good example is the hepatic portal circulation. Describe the purpose of this system in the box below.

The major blood vessels

Key Points:

1. Most major arteries arise from (branch off) the aorta, which runs from the heart to the pelvic region.
2. Most major veins drain into either the cranial or caudal vena cava depending on their positions in the body.
3. Smaller vessels branch from these major vessels.

List the structures

From reliable sources or during surgery, complete the following tables by writing in the names of the major arteries and veins that are found in each body region.

Arteries

Head and neck	*Thorax*	*Abdomen*	*Forelimbs*	*Hindlimbs*

Veins

Head and neck	*Thorax*	*Abdomen*	*Forelimbs*	*Hindlimbs*

What am I?

Exercise 7.13 Name the blood vessels described below, writing the correct answer in the box provided.

We are the vessels that supply the muscle of the heart.	(1)
I drain the intercostal region. I run through the thoracic cavity to empty into the junction of the vena cava and right atrium at a right angle.	(2)
I arise from the aorta in the abdomen and supply the liver, spleen and stomach.	(3)

(Continued)

I am the largest artery in the body.	(4)
I am the largest vein in the body.	(5)
I run from the small intestine to the liver. My purpose is to take absorbed nutrients directly to the liver.	(6)
I run down the hindlimb on the medial aspect. I am commonly used for pulse measurement.	(7)
I am a continuation of the axillary artery on the medial aspect of the proximal forelimb.	(8)
I arise from the brachiocephalic artery and run through the neck towards the head.	(9)
I am the only large superficial vein of the thoracic limb and lie on its dorsal aspect.	(10)

THE LYMPHATIC SYSTEM

Facts and functions of the lymphatic system

1. The prefix denoting the lymphatic system is *lymph–*.
2. The lymphatic system has several functions:
   a. to return tissue fluid and proteins back to the bloodstream
   b. to transport the products of fat digestion (in the form of *chylomicrons*)
   c. to filter bacteria and other harmful substances from the body's fluids
   d. to manufacture lymphocytes.

Fill in the gaps

Exercise 7.14 Complete the paragraph by filling in the gaps using the correct words from the selection below.

- small intestine
- fluid
- protein
- antigens
- fat
- macrophages
- proteins
- lacteals
- oedema
- interstitial
- lymphocytes
- bacteria

Fluid and smaller (1)__________ are constantly moving from the blood capillaries into the (2)__________ spaces. Although some fluid will move directly back into the capillaries, most will return via the lymphatic system; (3)__________ also returns via this route. This system enables the correct (4)__________ balance within the tissue spaces. If the lymphatic system does not function for some reason (5)__________ will occur in that particular body region.

Another substance transported via the lymphatic system to the bloodstream is digested (6)__________, which is absorbed through special lymphatic vessels in the (7)__________ wall called (8)__________. The lymphatic system also plays a part in body defence. In the lymph node foreign material, such as (9)__________, are prevented from continuing any further by the presence of phagocytic cells (10)(__________), which engulf and destroy them. Another function of the lymph node is to produce (11)__________, which leave the node in the lymph and eventually enter the bloodstream where they defend the body by reacting against (12)__________.

Lymph

Key Points:

1. Lymph is the name of the fluid circulating in the lymphatic system.
2. The composition of lymph is similar to that of blood plasma but lower in protein as the larger protein molecules cannot leave the blood capillaries. Lymph composition does change, however, in different parts of the body. For example:
   a. in the small intestinal region
   b. in the liver.
3. Lymph is usually clear and straw coloured. However, in the small intestinal region it takes on a cloudy appearance due to the high amount of fat present. Lymph in this state is known as *chyle*.

Lymphatic vessels

Key Points:

1. Unlike blood vessels, lymphatic vessels do not form a two-way system. They begin in the body tissues as a tiny mesh of lymph capillaries and slowly link up as they move towards the heart.
2. All lymph vessels eventually drain into one of two large lymphatic ducts—the *right lymphatic duct* or the *cisterna chyli* (called the thoracic duct as it runs through the thoracic region).
3. The lymphatic ducts drain into the cranial vena cava, near the right atrium, thus returning the fluid to the bloodstream.

Activity

Exercise 7.15 Fill in the chart below to describe the differences between lymph and blood vessels.

	Lymph vessels	Blood vessels
Number of capillaries in body tissues	(1)	(2)
Direction of transport in relation to the heart	(3)	(4)
Presence of valves along length	(5)	(6)
Presence of smooth muscle in vessel wall	(7)	(8)

Activity

Exercise 7.16 Complete the chart below by ticking the boxes to show which lymphatic duct drains each body region.

	Cisterna chyli/thoracic duct	Right lymphatic duct
Head and neck		
Right forelimb		

(Continued)

Left forelimb
Thorax
Abdomen
Right hindlimb
Left hindlimb

Lymph nodes

Key Points:

1. Lymph nodes are small round structures made up of lymphoid tissue and found interspersed throughout the lymphatic system.
2. Lymph flows through the lymph nodes on the way back to the bloodstream.
3. Macrophages in lymph nodes remove harmful contaminants, e.g. bacteria, from the lymph by phagocytosis.
4. Lymphocytes are produced in the lymph nodes from cells that originated in the myeloid tissue and are released into the lymph. They enter the bloodstream when the lymph drains into the cranial vena cava.

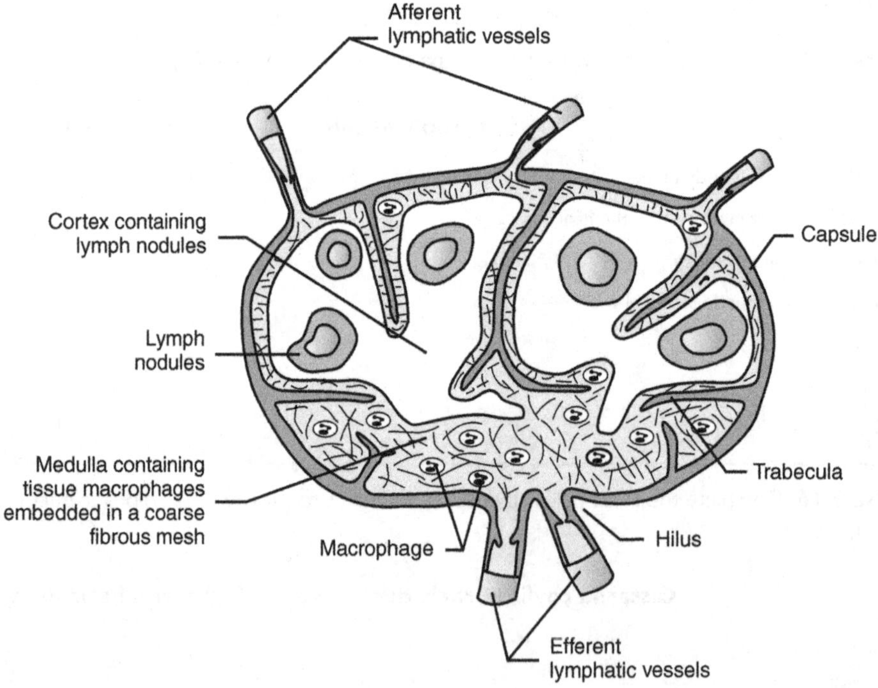

Figure 7.6 Cross-section through a lymph node.
(Reproduced with kind permission from Colville & Bassert 2002.)

Activity

Exercise 7.17 Draw and label the lymph nodes, as in the grid below, on the following diagram.

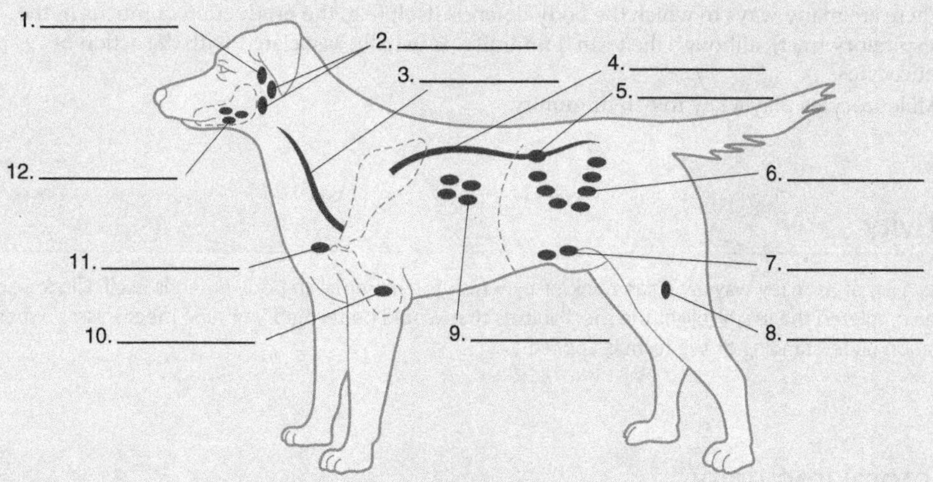

Mesenteric lymph nodes	Popliteal lymph node	Retropharyngeal lymph nodes	Axillary lymph node
Tracheal duct	Prescapular lymph node	Superficial inguinal lymph nodes	Parotid lymph node
Bronchial lymph nodes	Cisterna chyli	Submandibular lymph node	Thoracic duct

Figure 7.7 Diagram of the position of the lymph nodes in a dog.
(Reproduced with kind permission from CAW et al 2005.)

Other areas of lymph tissue

There are other areas of the body where lymphatic tissue is found.

Key Points:

1. Thymus; found in the mediastinum. The thymus is an important site for lymphocyte production in the juvenile animal but is largely replaced by fat in adulthood.
2. Tonsils; found in the tonsillar fossae on the lateral surfaces of the pharynx.
3. Spleen; found next to the stomach, the spleen also plays a part in erythrocyte storage and destruction.
4. Gut-associated lymphoid tissue (GALT); found in the small intestinal mucosa and also known as *Peyer's patches*.

THE IMMUNE SYSTEM

Facts and functions of the immune system

1. Immunity is the body's defence against harmful micro-organisms and their effects.
2. There are many ways in which the body defends itself (e.g. the production of mucus in the respiratory tract), although the term 'immunity' is usually associated with the action of leucocytes.
3. All leucocytes play a key role in immunity.

Activity

Make a list of as many ways you can think of by which the mammalian body defends itself. Once you have completed the list, highlight the mechanisms that would be termed 'immune mechanisms' when the common understanding of the term is applied.

Humoral immunity

Key Points:

1. Humoral immunity occurs within the fluid of the body, i.e. within the bloodstream, a body cavity or mucosal surface.
2. This type of immunity comprises mechanisms involving soluble substances, namely immunoglobulins (otherwise known as antibodies).
3. Immunoglobulins are proteins produced by a type of lymphocyte called a B-lymphocyte.
4. B-lymphocytes are derived from the myeloid tissue, then move to the lymphatic tissue and eventually mature in the bloodstream where they are called plasma cells.
5. Immunoglobulins are produced in response to invasion by foreign matter—the antigen.

Fill in the gaps

Exercise 7.18 Complete the paragraphs on humoral immunity by filling in the gaps using the correct words from the selection below.

- antigen
- antiserum
- antibodies
- colostrum
- virus
- active
- passive
- vaccine
- plasma cell

Humoral immunity is the type of immunity involving immunoglobulins, or (1)____________. These are proteins produced by a type of lymphocyte, known as a B-lymphocyte, which matures into a (2)____________. Antibodies are produced in response to invasion by foreign matter, e.g. bacteria or a (3)____________. The invading matter is called the (4)____________. Each antibody

(Continued)

is specific to the antigen that triggered its production and is not effective against other antigens. Antibodies work in a number of ways. They 'bind' to the foreign matter to prevent it damaging the body's cells; they make phagocytosis easier and also initiate the inflammatory response.

When antibodies are produced by the body in response to antigens, the immunity that results is called (5)______________; a (6)______________ works on this principle. If an animal is actually given the antibodies, the immunity that results is called (7)______________; (8)______________ works on this principle. The immunity that results from the newborn animal taking its mother's (9)______________ is also passive.

Cellular immunity

Key Points:

1. Cellular immunity involves a certain type of lymphocyte derived from the myeloid tissue but maturing in the thymus; this is called a T-lymphocyte. See section entitled 'Leucocytes' in this chapter for further general information about lymphocytes.
2. T-lymphocytes combine with antigens and act in two ways:
   a. they produce special substances called lymphokines. These attract phagocytic cells to the antigen and also initiate the inflammatory response
   b. they damage the harmful micro-organisms as they combine with them.

Phagocytosis

Key Points:

1. Phagocytosis is the process by which certain cells engulf and destroy harmful particles in the body.
2. The two main phagocytic cells are neutrophils and macrophages.
3. Neutrophils are the main type of lymphocyte in the blood of dogs and cats.
4. Macrophages are found at various sites in the body. They are sometimes given different names:
   a. monocytes in the bloodstream
   b. Kupffer cells in the liver
   c. histiocytes in the connective tissue.
5. The macrophage system is sometimes called the mononuclear phagocytic system or the reticuloendothelial system.

Activity

Design a poster on A3 paper depicting the process of phagocytosis. Use large labels and bold colours. When you have finished, stick it up where you will regularly read it. Why not on a kitchen cupboard?

General revision

What am I?

Exercise 7.19 Name the structures described below, writing the correct answer in the space provided.

I am a blood vessel that drains into the right atrium.	(1)
I am a valve comprising two cusps; my other name is 'mitral'.	(2)
I am the structure separating the left and right sides of the heart; in the fetus I am incomplete.	(3)
I am the chamber that blood leaves as it enters the aorta.	(4)
I am the vessel taking the blood to the lungs for oxygenation.	(5)
I am the fetal blood vessel that allows blood to bypass the pulmonary circulation.	(6)
I am the opposite end to the heart's base.	(7)
I make up the outer layer of the myocardium and the innermost layer of the pericardium.	(8)
I am the pacemaker of the heart.	(9)
I am the pressure wave within an artery caused by contraction of the left ventricle.	(10)

Multiple choice questions – the heart

Exercise 7.20

1. The heart is positioned on the:
   a. right side of the thorax tilting dorsocranially
   b. left side of the thorax tilting ventrocaudally
   c. right side of the thorax tilting ventrocaudally
   d. left side of the thorax tilting dorsocranially.
2. The innermost layer of the myocardium, which also forms the cusps of the valves, is the:
   a. endocardium
   b. Purkinje tissue
   c. epicardium
   d. pulmonary tissue.
3. The valve situated between the right atrium and right ventricle is the:
   a. bicuspid valve
   b. aortic semilunar valve
   c. tricuspid valve
   d. pulmonary semilunar valve.

4. The fibromuscular cords, which run from the papillary muscles to the atrioventricular valves, are the:
   a. myofibrils
   b. chordae tendinae
   c. microfibres
   d. chorda tympani.
5. On leaving the right ventricle, blood moves into the:
   a. coronary artery
   b. pulmonary artery
   c. coronary vein
   d. pulmonary vein.
6. Before entering the right atrium, blood is in the:
   a. vena cava
   b. jugular vein
   c. aorta
   d. pulmonary circulation.
7. Blood pressure is regulated by both the:
   a. nervous and endocrine systems
   b. pulmonary and nervous systems
   c. urinary and endocrine systems
   d. endocrine and pulmonary systems.
8. Systole causes:
   a. emptying of corresponding heart chambers
   b. inhalation of air
   c. filling of corresponding heart chambers
   d. exhalation of air.

Tip: *Why not get together with fellow students and write some more questions for each other?*

Multiple choice questions – the blood vascular system

Exercise 7.21

1. The pH of blood is approximately:
   a. 4.4
   b. 4.7
   c. 7.4
   d. 7.7.
2. The plasma protein responsible for maintaining the osmotic pressure of blood is:
   a. albumin
   b. keratin
   c. fibrin
   d. myosin.

3. Approximately how many millions of erythrocytes are there per microlitre of blood?
   a. 1
   b. 3
   c. 7
   d. 9.
4. Which of the following leucocytes is agranular?
   a. neutrophil
   b. monocyte
   c. basophil
   d. eosinophil.
5. The leucocyte that is the most numerous in canine and feline blood is the:
   a. lymphocyte
   b. basophil
   c. monocyte
   d. neutrophil.
6. In the fetus, the pulmonary artery and aorta are linked by the:
   a. foramen ovale
   b. ductus arteriosus
   c. falciform ligament
   d. umbilical vein.
7. The organs supplied by end arteries are the:
   a. liver, kidney and spleen
   b. brain, heart and spleen
   c. liver, kidney and brain
   d. brain, heart and kidney.
8. The hepatic portal vein runs between the:
   a. small intestine and liver
   b. heart and spleen
   c. small intestine and heart
   d. spleen and liver.
9. Which of the following vessels is often used for blood collection?
   a. hepatic artery
   b. jugular vein
   c. carotid artery
   d. renal vein.
10. The part of the vascular system where blood is oxygenated is the:
    a. systemic circulation
    b. fetal circulation
    c. pulmonary circulation
    d. portal circulation.

Tip: *Why not get together with fellow students and write some more questions for each other?*

Word chart

Exercise 7.22

	L	E												I
	E		R		N						A			M
	U			Y	U		L				E			M
	C		S		T		H				R			U
	O		E		R	H	A	A	L	B	U	M	I	N
	C		T		I		R						W	O
	Y		Y		E		T	O					A	G
	T		C		N		C		C				T	L
	E		O		T		L			Y			E	O
	S		B		S		M				T		R	B
	E		M									E		U
	B	H	O	R	M	O	N	E	S				S	L
	U		R											I
	I		H											N
C	L	O	T	T	I	N	G	F	A	C	T	O	R	S

Clues

1. A small vein found within the body organ it supplies.
2. An unpaired vein emptying into the junction of the right atrium and vena cava.
3. Plasma without the clotting factors.
4. Vessel supplying the heart muscle.
5. A waste product of protein breakdown excreted by the kidney.
6. An agranular leucocyte with a large nucleus occupying most of the cell.
7. The largest artery in the body.
8. The vena cavae drain into this heart chamber.
9. Another term for immunoglobulins.
10. The organ that produces renin.
11. Term meaning erythrocyte production.
12. The end-product of the coagulation cascade.
13. A platelet.
14. The dividing wall in the heart separating oxygenated and deoxygenated blood.

Multiple choice questions – the lymphatic system

Exercise 7.23

1. When compared with blood plasma, lymph:
   a. has a lower protein content
   b. has a slightly higher protein content
   c. has the same protein content
   d. has a much higher protein content.
2. The term used for lymph present in the lacteals is:
   a. chyle
   b. intestinal juice
   c. chyme
   d. gastric juice.
3. Peyer's patches are found in the:
   a. tonsils
   b. intestine
   c. thymus
   d. lacteals.
4. The lymph node situated on the caudal aspect of the thigh is the:
   a. inguinal
   b. parotid
   c. axillary
   d. popliteal.
5. Lymph in the lymphatic ducts drains into the:
   a. lymphatic vessels
   b. cranial vena cava
   c. lymph nodes
   d. caudal vena cava.

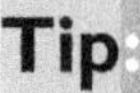

Why not get together with fellow students and write some more questions for each other?

Multiple choice questions – the immune system

Exercise 7.24

1. A mature B-lymphocyte is called a:
   a. phagocyte
   b. macrophage
   c. plasma cell
   d. lymphokine.
2. T-lymphocytes mature in the:
   a. myeloid tissue
   b. thymus
   c. lymph nodes
   d. bloodstream.

3. Immunoglobulins are also called:
   a. antigens
   b. antisera
   c. antibodies
   d. antitoxins.
4. An example of passive immunity is:
   a. vaccination with a live vaccine
   b. actually catching the disease
   c. obtaining the mother's colostrum
   d. vaccination with a killed vaccine.
5. Which of the following is not phagocytic?
   a. monocyte
   b. neutrophil
   c. basophil
   d. histiocyte.

Tip: *Why not get together with fellow students and write some more questions for each other?*

CHAPTER 8

The respiratory system

LEARNING Objectives

This chapter will help you to revise the following:

- facts and functions of the respiratory system
- the nose, nasal cavity and paranasal sinuses
- the pharynx and larynx
- the trachea, bronchi and bronchioles
- the alveoli and gaseous exchange
- the lungs and associated structures
- breathing.

There is a general revision section at the end of this chapter.

Facts and functions of the respiratory system

1. All mammals have respiratory systems, which are used in a similar way, involving the exchange of the gases oxygen and carbon dioxide by use of lung tissue.
2. Other functions of the respiratory system are:
   a. panting to control temperature by evaporation
   b. phonation (barking in dogs and mewing in cats)
   c. purring in cats, an action that involves both the diaphragm and the larynx.
3. The respiratory tract is protected in several ways:
   a. most of the tract is lined with mucous epithelium, which aids the expulsion of foreign matter
   b. the nasal cavity filters air on inhalation
   c. the larynx protects the lower respiratory tract
   d. the cough reflex.
4. The prefix *pulmo–* pertains to the lungs.
5. The prefix *pneumo–* pertains to air.
6. The suffix *–pnoea* pertains to breathing.

Fill in the gaps

Exercise 8.1 Complete the paragraph by filling in the gaps using the correct words from the selection below.

- environment
- body tissues
- gases
- adenosine triphosphate
- bloodstream
- oxygen
- carbon dioxide
- lungs
- carbon dioxide

Respiration is essential for survival. Respiration involves the exchange of (1)__________, or 'gaseous exchange', in this case (2)__________ and (3)__________. External respiration is gaseous exchange between an animal and its (4)__________ and occurs in the (5)__________. Internal respiration is gaseous exchange between the (6)__________ and (7)__________. Oxygen is necessary in order for the body's cells to obtain energy in the form of (8)__________ (ATP). An end-product of this process is the production of (9)__________, which needs to be removed from the cells.

The nose, nasal cavity and paranasal sinuses

Key Points:

1. The main function of the nose, nasal cavity and paranasal sinuses is to prepare inhaled air before it moves down to the lower respiratory tract. This means warming, filtering and moistening the air.
2. Surface area is maximized by the presence of the scrolled turbinate bones and the paranasal sinuses.
3. A ciliated mucous epithelium lining allows filtering and moistening to occur.

Link the words

Exercise 8.2 Match the description in the left-hand column to the correct definition in the right-hand column by drawing a line to link them.

(1) The structure dividing the nasal cavity into left and right sides	(2) Frontal
(3) The turbinate bones are lined with this tissue	(4) Alar fold
(5) Another term for the nostrils	(6) Ethmoid
(7) The bone containing a large paranasal sinus	(8) Ciliated columnar epithelium
(9) The bone separating the nasal and cranial cavities	(10) Nasal septum
(11) The structure separating the nasal and oral cavities	(12) Elastic cartilage
(13) A flap of cartilage forming a protective bulb just inside the nostril	(14) Hard palate
(15) The bulk of the rhinarium is made from this tissue	(16) Nares

The pharynx and larynx

Key Points:

1. The pharynx is divided into two parts:
   a. the nasopharynx situated behind the nasal cavity
   b. the oropharynx situated behind the oral cavity.
2. The pharynx is shared with the digestive tract (see Ch. 9, 'The Digestive System', for more information).
3. The larynx is situated between the pharynx and the trachea and is suspended from the base of the skull by the bony hyoid apparatus; this has the ability to swing so that movement in the neck is not restricted.

4. The larynx comprises six rigid hyaline cartilage structures held together to form a hole through their centre (the glottis).
5. The epiglottis is a cartilage that forms a 'lid' over the glottis during deglutition; this can be seen during endotracheal intubation.
6. On each side of the larynx, projecting from the arytenoid cartilage is the vocal fold. Each vocal fold contains a vocal ligament made up of several elastic fibres (the vocal cords).
7. The vocal cords are responsible for phonation, i.e. sound production.

Mnemonic

To remember the functions of the larynx.
The three Ps:

Passage of air
Protection of the respiratory tract
Phonation (sound production)

List the structures

Exercise 8.3 List the names of the laryngeal cartilages in the space below.

The trachea, bronchi and bronchioles

Key Points:

1. Along the length of the trachea is a series of incomplete cartilage rings; these allow it to maintain its rigid and patent structure.
2. Between each of the tracheal rings is an annular ligament, made up of fibrous connective tissue and smooth muscle.
3. The trachea runs from the larynx to just above the heart, where it divides (bifurcates) to become two principal bronchi (singular, bronchus).
4. Each bronchus then branches into smaller bronchi, which then become the even smaller bronchioles.
5. These bronchioles also branch into yet smaller and thinner bronchioles.
6. The last bronchiole in each branch is called the terminal bronchiole.
7. The trachea, bronchi and bronchioles all have a mucoid epithelial lining, which protects the lower respiratory tract by moving foreign particles upwards towards the pharynx where they can be coughed out.

Activity

Exercise 8.4 In the following diagram of the trachea and bronchi, add the correct labels from the selection below.

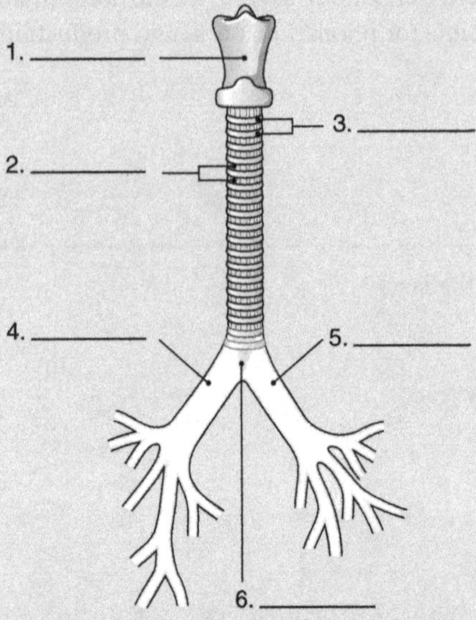

Bifurcation of the trachea	Hyaline cartilage rings	Right principal bronchus
Annular ligaments	Left principal bronchus	Larynx

Figure 8.1 Diagram of the trachea and bronchi.
(Adapted with kind permission from Reece 1997.)

Activity

Examine some radiographs of dogs and cats. Which is more ventral, the trachea or the oesophagus?

The alveoli and gaseous exchange

Key Points:

1. Each terminal bronchus narrows down into a small duct (the alveolar duct).
2. Each alveolar duct leads to an alveolar sac, from which branch several alveoli (singular, alveolus).

3. Alveoli are lined by the pulmonary membrane, which is made of simple squamous epithelial tissue. Tiny capillaries surround each alveolus.
4. It is in the alveoli that gaseous exchange occurs between the animal and its environment (external respiration).

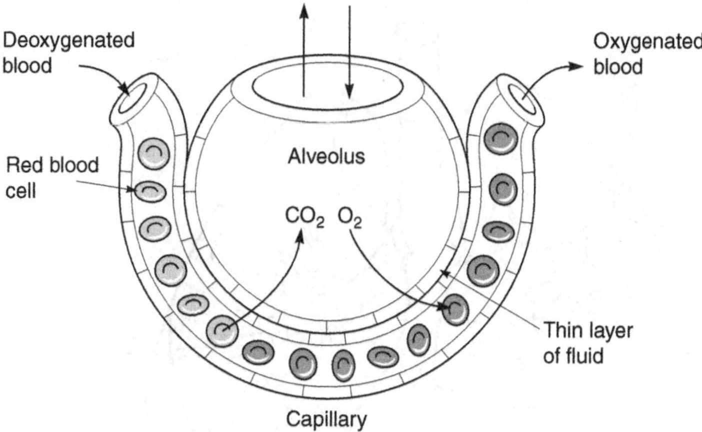

Figure 8.2 Diagram of gaseous exchange between an alveolus and a blood capillary.
(Reproduced with kind permission from Bowden & Masters 2001.)

The lungs and associated structures

Key Points:

1. There are two lungs, one on each side of the thoracic cavity.
2. Each lung comprises the bronchial tree and respiratory surfaces, i.e. the bronchi, bronchioles and alveoli.
3. Each lung is divided into a number of lobes:
   a. cranial or apical
   b. middle or cardiac
   c. caudal or diaphragmatic
   d. the right lung has a fourth lobe, the accessory lobe.
4. The pulmonary artery and vein, principal bronchus, nerves and lymphatic vessels of each lung enter and leave at the hilus.
5. The thoracic cavity is divided into left and right pleural cavities by the mediastinum.
6. The lungs, thoracic cavity, mediastinum and diaphragm are lined with a serous membrane (the pleura) which prevents friction caused by movement.

Activity

Exercise 8.5 In the following diagram of the lungs, add the correct labels from the selection below.

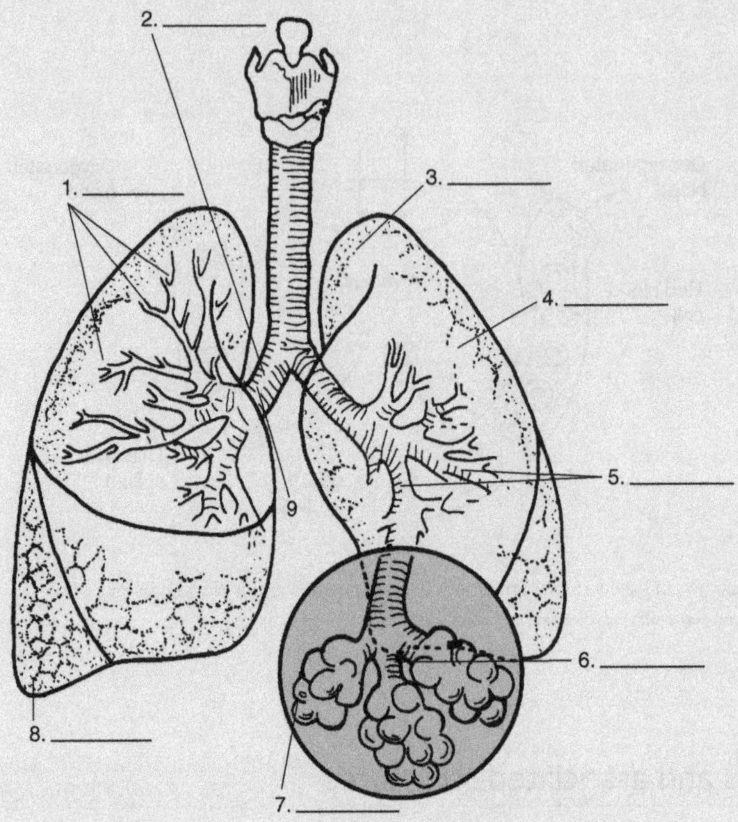

Principal bronchus	Bronchi	Hilus	Alveolus	Cardiac lobe
Accessory lobe	Bronchioles	Alveolar duct	Apical lobe	

Figure 8.3 Diagram of the lungs.
(Reproduced with kind permission from Colville & Bassert 2002.)

List the structures

Exercise 8.6 List the structures contained within the mediastinum:

Breathing

Key Points:

1. Breathing involves the inhalation of air into the lungs through the nose (and sometimes the mouth) and the exhalation of air via the same route(s).
2. The purpose of breathing is to conduct air to the respiratory surfaces, namely the alveoli.
3. Respiratory rate is affected by many things but is ultimately controlled by three respiratory centres in the medulla and pons of the brain.

The action of breathing

Inhalation The diaphragm and intercostal muscles contract together. The ribs move outwards and the diaphragm flattens. This increases the volume of the thoracic cavity. The lungs then expand and the pressure within them is less than the pressure outside, hence air is sucked in.
Exhalation The diaphragm and intercostal muscles relax, thoracic volume decreases and the lungs contract, which forces air out.

Look it up

Exercise 8.7 Complete the chart by writing in the percentages of gases that make up air.

Component	Inhaled air	Exhaled air
Nitrogen	(1)	(2)
Oxygen	(3)	(4)
Carbon dioxide	(5)	(6)
Water vapour	Variable	Increased by comparison
Other gases	Trace	Trace

Link the words

Exercise 8.8 Match the description in the left-hand column to the correct definition in the right-hand column by drawing a line to link them.

(1)The air that is breathed in and out during normal respiration	(2)Total lung capacity
(3)The amount of air that is breathed in. Usually measured in mL/kg	(4)Residual volume
(5)The amount of air needed to fill every part of the lung	(6)Tidal air
(7)The amount of air that can be expired	(8)Anatomical dead space
(9)The air left in the lungs after forced exhalation	(10)Functional residual capacity
(11)The area of the respiratory tract not used for gaseous exchange	(12)Vital capacity
(13)The air left in the lungs after normal exhalation which allows gaseous exchange to continue	(14)Tidal volume

Activity

Exercise 8.9 Write the normal respiratory rates for dogs and cats in the spaces below.

Dog
Cat

There are many factors that can affect respiratory rate. Write some down.

General revision

Multiple choice questions

Exercise 8.10

1. The turbinate bones are lined with:
   a. elastic cartilage
   b. ciliated columnar epithelium
   c. hyaline cartilage
   d. simple squamous epithelium.
2. The groove between the nares is called the:
   a. philtrum
   b. septum
   c. rhinarium
   d. epithelium.
3. The pharynx is separated by the:
   a. hard palate
   b. nasal septum
   c. soft palate
   d. cribriform plate.
4. The annular ligament is made of:
   a. bone tissue and fibrocartilage
   b. fibrous connective tissue and smooth muscle
   c. striated muscle and hyaline cartilage
   d. ciliated columnar epithelium.
5. The bone that partially houses a sinus formed at the caudal end of each nasal chamber is the:
   a. frontal
   b. maxilla
   c. mandible
   d. occipital.
6. The trachea bifurcates:
   a. at the larynx
   b. just above the heart
   c. just below the heart
   d. at the lung hilus.

7. The pulmonary membrane lines the:
   a. pharynx
   b. thoracic cavity
   c. lung
   d. alveoli.
8. The upper respiratory tract comprises the:
   a. nose and nasal cavity only
   b. nose, nasal cavity and the pharynx only
   c. nose, nasal cavity, pharynx and larynx only
   d. nose, nasal cavity, pharynx, larynx and trachea.
9. The accessory lobe is found on the:
   a. left bronchus
   b. left lung
   c. right bronchus
   d. right lung.
10. Which laryngeal cartilage prevents food moving into the larynx?
    a. arytenoid
    b. epiglottis
    c. crichoid
    d. thyroid.
11. The muscles involved in normal respiration are the:
    a. diaphragm and intercostal muscles
    b. abdominal oblique and pectoral muscles
    c. intercostal and pectoral muscles
    d. intercostal and abdominal oblique muscles.
12. Tidal volume is:
    a. 1–5 ml/kg
    b. 10–15 ml/kg
    c. 100–150 ml/kg
    d. 1–5 l/kg.
13. Bradypnoea is:
    a. abnormally fast breathing
    b. difficult breathing
    c. abnormally slow breathing
    d. absence of breathing.
14. Which of the following structures is not contained in the mediastinum?
    a. lungs
    b. heart
    c. oesophagus
    d. thymus.
15. The pleura is the:
    a. first lobe of the lung
    b. smallest laryngeal cartilage
    c. serous lining of the thoracic cavity
    d. membrane across which gaseous exchange occurs.
16. Pulmonary oedema is:
    a. accumulation of fluid in the lung tissue
    b. accumulation of air in the lung tissue
    c. absence of air in the lung tissue
    d. absence of fluid in the lung tissue.

17. The parts of the respiratory tract inside the thoracic cavity are the:
    a. nasal cavity, pharynx and larynx
    b. pharynx, larynx and trachea
    c. larynx, trachea, bronchi and bronchial tree
    d. pharynx, trachea, bronchi and bronchial tree.
18. Residual volume is approximately:
    a. 1% of total lung capacity
    b. 20% of total lung capacity
    c. 50% of total lung capacity
    d. 70% of total lung capacity.

Tip: *Why not get together with fellow students and write some more questions for each other?*

Word chart

Exercise 8.11

1	R													
2	E													
3	S													
4	P													
5	I													
6	R													
7	A													
8	T													
9	I													
10	O													
11	N													

Clues

1. The air left in the lung after forced exhalation.
2. The bone separating the nasal and cranial cavities.
3. The pleura is this type of lining.
4. The artery that supplies the lung with deoxygenated blood.
5. A small laryngeal cartilage.
6. Hering-Breuer is one of these.
7. The extra lobe on the right lung.
8. The scrolls of bone in the nasal cavity are called this.
9. The process of breathing in.
10. The tube that sits dorsally to the trachea.
11. The nostrils.

Tip: *Have you seen a word you don't understand? Don't ignore it, look it up!*

CHAPTER 9

The digestive system

LEARNING Objectives

This chapter will help you to revise the following:

- facts and functions of the digestive system
- the oral cavity
- the teeth
- the pharynx
- the oesophagus
- the stomach
- the small intestine
- the large intestine
- the pancreas
- the liver and gall bladder
- the physiology of digestion
- digestive enzymes
- faeces and defecation.

There is a general revision section at the end of the chapter.

Facts and functions of the digestive system

1. The digestive system is the means by which an animal digests and absorbs nutrients from food, without which it would not be able to sustain life.
2. The gastrointestinal (GI) tract and associated structures comprise the digestive system.
3. The digestive system of an animal is adapted to suit its diet, so they do vary significantly between some species. However, the digestive systems of dogs and cats are similar.
4. Essentially, the GI tract is a hollow tube running from the mouth to the anus.

Study

Consider the diets of dogs, cats, rabbits, horses and cattle. How do they differ? Find out how their GI tracts differ.

The oral cavity

Key Points:

1. The oral cavity is the entrance to the GI tract and is lined with stratified squamous mucous epithelium.
2. The oral cavity comprises two main parts:
   a. the oral vestibule, which is situated between the lips, cheeks (buccae) and teeth
   b. the true oral cavity, which is situated between the teeth and the pharynx.
3. The dorsal surface comprises the hard palate, which separates the oral and nasal cavities.
4. There are four pairs of salivary glands whose ducts open into the oral cavity.
5. The tongue is connected to the ventral surface of the oral cavity by the lingual frenulum, although its base (root) is in the pharynx.

Activity

Exercise 9.1 The following diagram is a dog's head. From the selection below, add the labels to the diagram.

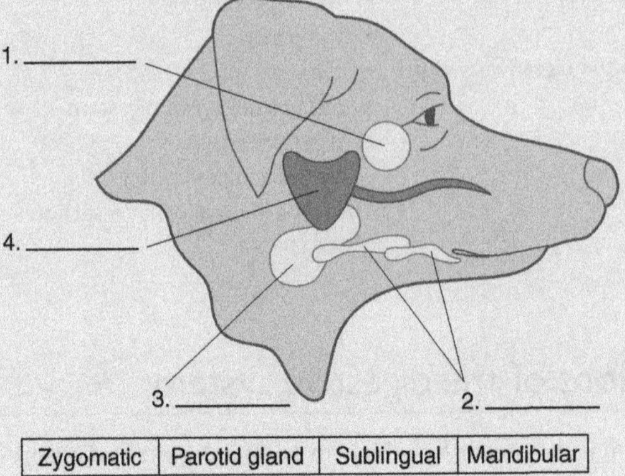

Zygomatic	Parotid gland	Sublingual	Mandibular

Figure 9.1 Diagram of the positions of the salivary glands.
(Reproduced with kind permission from CAW et al 2005.)

List the structures

Exercise 9.2 The tongue is a highly muscular organ with several functions. List them below:

The teeth

Key Points:

1. Dogs and cats have two sets of teeth in their lifetime.
2. The deciduous (milk) dentition erupts at around four weeks of age.
3. The permanent dentition erupts at around four months of age, replacing the shed deciduous teeth.
4. Each tooth sits in a socket (alveolar cavity) and is attached by the fibrous periodontal ligament.
5. Dogs and cats have four different types of teeth, each designed to perform a different function:
   a. incisors (very small teeth designed to hold prey)
   b. canines (the long 'fang' or 'eye' teeth designed to hold and kill prey)
   c. premolars and molars (designed for shearing and stripping meat from carcasses).
   There are no molars in the deciduous dentition.
6. The last upper premolar is a large triple-rooted tooth known as the carnassial.
7. The number of teeth in an animal's mouth is recorded in a standard way—this is known as the dental formula.

Activity

Exercise 9.3 In the following diagram of a tooth add the correct labels to the diagram from the selection below.

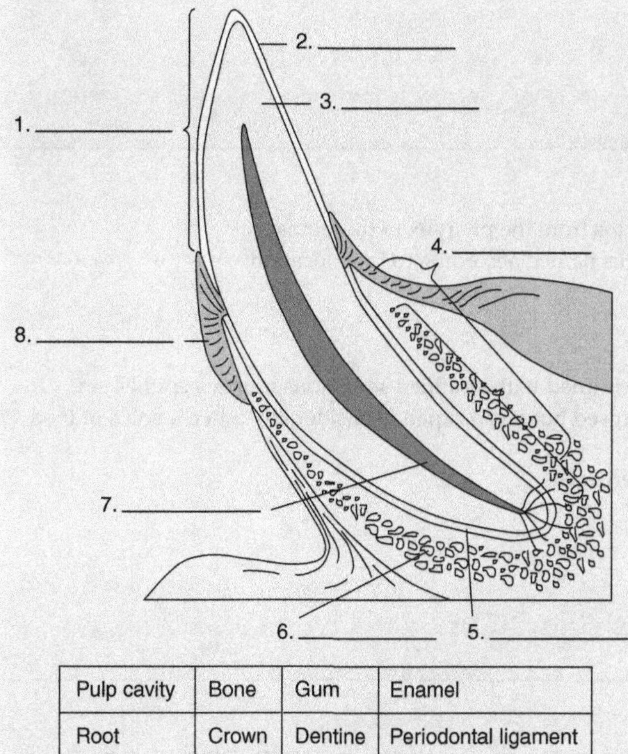

Pulp cavity	Bone	Gum	Enamel
Root	Crown	Dentine	Periodontal ligament

Figure 9.2 Cross-section of a typical animal tooth.

(Reproduced with kind permission from Colville & Bassert 2002.)

Tip: *Look at the shapes of teeth after extraction and on radiographs. Relate their shape to their function.*

The pharynx

Key Points:

1. The pharynx is shared with the GI and respiratory tracts.
2. The pharynx is separated into two sections by the soft palate:
   a. the nasopharynx, which is found directly behind the nasal cavity
   b. the oropharynx, which is found directly behind the oral cavity.
3. On the lateral surfaces (fauces) of the pharynx are areas of lymphoid tissue—the tonsils. Each one is usually hidden from view as it sits in a hollow—the tonsillar fossa.

List the structures

Exercise 9.4 There are many structures adjacent or leading to or from the pharynx. Make a list of them.

The oesophagus

Key Points:

1. This tube, made largely of muscle, runs from the pharynx to the stomach.
2. There are three sections of oesophagus named according to their location:
   a. cervical
   b. thoracic
   c. abdominal.
3. The inner surface of the oesophagus is lined with stratified squamous mucous epithelium.
4. When empty the oesophagus is collapsed but it can expand considerably when a bolus of food moves through it.
5. Food boluses are moved along by peristalsis.

The stomach

Key Points:

1. Positioned in the cranial abdominal cavity, the stomach lies transversally and to the left on the sagittal plane, near the liver.
2. The stomach is essentially a large muscular sac leading from the oesophagus to the small intestine.
3. The inner surface of the stomach contains many mucus-producing goblet cells and glands producing digestive enzymes.
4. The inner surface sits in large folds that allow the stomach to expand considerably.
5. The three main functions of the stomach are:
   a. the mechanical and chemical digestion of food
   b. storage of food
   c. control of the rate of release of food into the small intestine.
6. The cardiac sphincter prevents reflux of food—this must open in order to allow the animal to vomit.
7. The pyloric sphincter controls the release of matter into the small intestine—it does this over a period of 2–4 hours.

Activity

Exercise 9.5 In the following diagram of a stomach, add the correct labels to the diagram from the selection below.

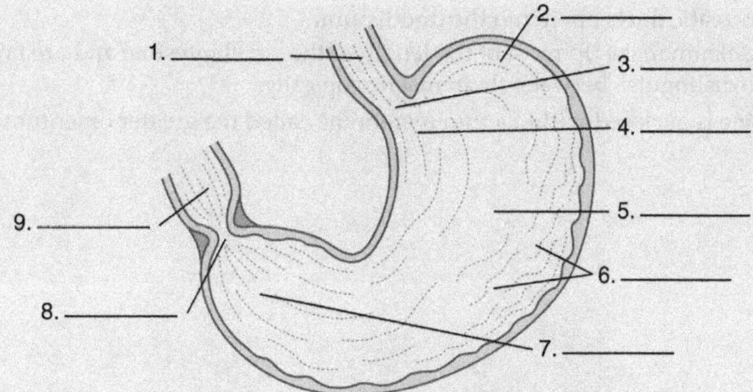

Pyloric sphincter	Oesophagus	Pyloric antrum	Fundus	Duodenum
Body	Rugae	Cardia	Oesophageal (cardiac) sphincter	

Figure 9.3 Diagram of the stomach.
(Reproduced with kind permission from CAW et al 2005.)

Study

Exercise 9.6 Write a paragraph explaining the differences between regurgitation and vomiting.

The small intestine

Key Points:

1. In the small intestine, chemical digestion continues and absorption of digested food products occurs.
2. The small intestine has three parts:
   a. the duodenum
   b. the jejunum
   c. the ileum
3. The small intestinal wall contains smooth muscle capable of moving matter by peristalsis.

4. The inner lining of the small intestine comprises columnar epithelium interspersed with mucus-producing goblet cells and glands producing digestive enzymes.
5. The surface area of the small intestine is greatly increased as it is arranged in longitudinal folds and also has tiny projections on its inner surface—intestinal villi.
6. Each villus has a network of capillaries and a specialized lymph vessel (lacteal); these absorb digested food products.
7. The bile and pancreatic ducts open into the duodenum.
8. The jejunum and ileum make up most of the length of the small intestine and are fairly mobile; it is not possible to distinguish between them macroscopically.
9. The small intestine is enclosed within a thin membrane called the greater omentum.

Mnemonic

The ileum of the small intestine must not be confused with the ilium of the pelvis. A way of remembering the two is:

I for 'ips (hips) and E for eat

Activity

Exercise 9.7 In the following diagram of a cross-section through the small intestinal wall, add the correct labels from the selection below.

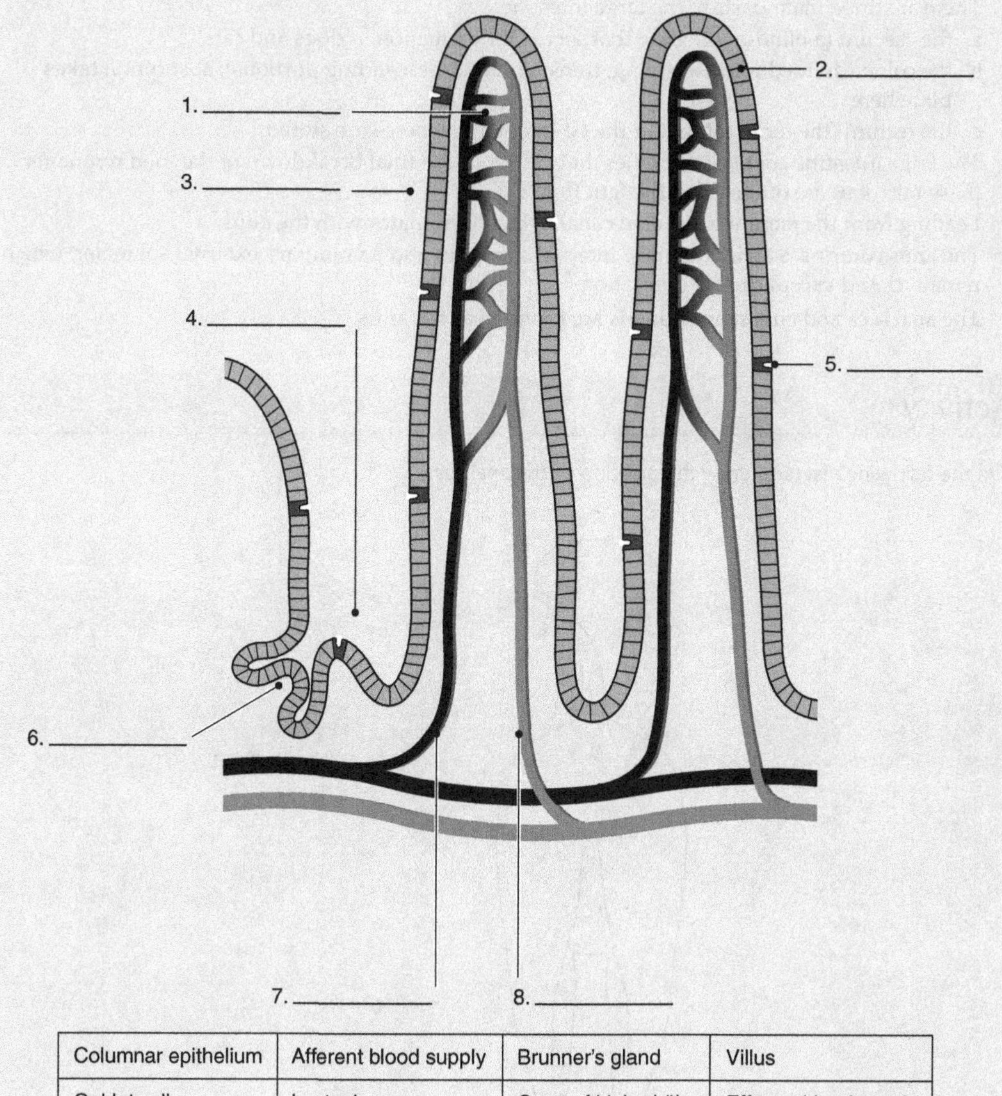

Columnar epithelium	Afferent blood supply	Brunner's gland	Villus
Goblet cell	Lacteal	Crypt of Lieberkühn	Efferent blood supply

Figure 9.4 Diagram of the small intestinal wall.

The large intestine

Key Points:

1. The large intestine serves to absorb water, electrolytes and water-soluble vitamins.
2. There are three main parts to the large intestine:
   a. the caecum (a blind-ending sac that serves little function in dogs and cats)
   b. the colon (divided into ascending, transverse and descending portions); absorption takes place here
   c. the rectum (the terminal part of the GI tract where faeces are stored).
3. The large intestine contains microbes that carry out the final breakdown of the food remnants; these microbes are often called the 'gut flora'.
4. Leading from the rectum is the anal canal, which terminates with the anus.
5. The anus comprises an involuntary internal sphincter and a voluntary external sphincter, which remain closed except during defecation.
6. The anal sacs and circumanal glands are found near the anus.

Activity

On the following diagram, draw the position of the anal sacs.

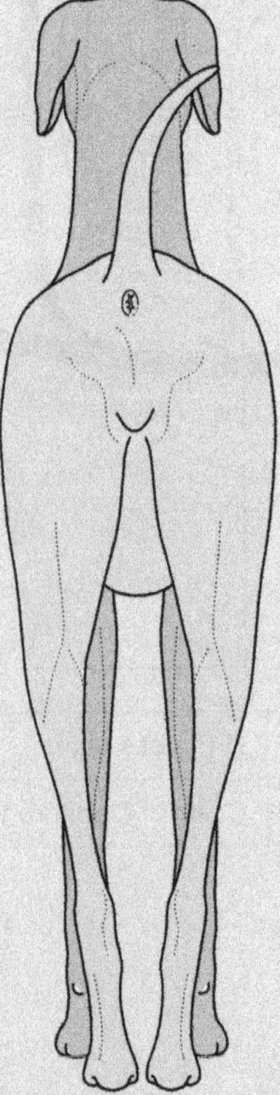

Figure 9.5 Position of the anal sacs.
(Adapted with kind permission from Boyd 2001.)

The pancreas

Key Points:

1. The pancreas is a lobed, greyish-pink, V-shaped organ situated alongside the stomach and duodenum.
2. The pancreas is a *mixed gland*, meaning it has both endocrine and exocrine functions.
3. The endocrine part of the pancreas produces several hormones (see Ch.6, 'The Endocrine System', for more information).
4. The exocrine part of the pancreas produces alkaline pancreatic juice, which enters the duodenum via two pancreatic ducts.

Study

Research the following two diseases:

- pancreatitis
- exocrine pancreatic insufficiency.

Consider the clinical symptoms of these diseases and why they occur. This will help you to understand the function of the pancreas.

The liver and gall bladder

Key Points:

1. The glandular liver is the largest organ in the abdominal cavity.
2. The liver is situated just caudal to the diaphragm, alongside the stomach.
3. A red–brown lobed organ, the liver is made from cubical epithelium and connective tissue among other cells, e.g. Kupffer cells.
4. The liver is held in place by several soft tissue ligaments; one, the falciform ligament, runs from the liver to the diaphragm, ventral abdominal wall and umbilicus. In the fetus, it carries the umbilical vein.
5. Blood enters the liver either from the hepatic artery or via the hepatic portal system.
6. The hepatic portal system enables nutrients to be transported directly to the liver from the small intestine.
7. The gall bladder is tucked between the lobes of the liver. It is a pear-shaped sac that stores bile and delivers it to the small intestine via the common bile duct.

Activity

The liver is the 'chemical factory' of the body. It is responsible for storing, detoxifying and producing many substances. Design a poster of liver functions on a piece of A3 paper. Use large labels and bold colours. When it is complete, stick it where you will regularly read it. Why not on a kitchen cupboard?

Table 9.1 Some of the functions of the liver

Storage of:	**Metabolism** of:
• glucose in the form of glycogen	• protein
• fat and fat-soluble vitamins	• fat
• iron	• carbohydrate
Production of:	**Detoxification** of:
• heat	• ammonia (by converting it into urea)
• bile	• any ingested posions
• plasma proteins	• many other substances

The physiology of digestion

Key Points:

1. There are two types of digestion:
   a. mechanical—this is where food is physically broken down by the action of teeth or muscles
   b. chemical—this is where food is broken down by the action of enzymes found in various parts of the GI tract.
2. Mechanical digestion begins in the oral cavity.
3. Chemical digestion begins in the stomach.

Activity

Exercise 9.8 Photocopy (or copy) the following digestive processes chart onto a large piece of paper and cut out each individual statement. Arrange the statements in the order in which they occur.

(1)The cardiac sphincter opens and food enters the stomach.

(2)The food bolus is then pushed to the pharynx by the tongue. The action of swallowing (deglutition) occurs by a combination of voluntary and reflex activity. The result is the epiglottis occludes the glottis and food moves into the oesophagus.

(3)The food mixed with gastric juice and mucus produces a paste known as chyme.

(4)Faecal matter is stored in the rectum until the animal is ready to pass it through the anus via the anal canal.

(5)In the duodenum, the environment turns from acid to slightly alkaline by the presence of bicarbonate.

(6)Food is taken into the oral cavity using the jaws and teeth (prehension).

(7)As the digestive process completes, the digested food products are absorbed through the intestinal villi into the blood and lymphatic systems.

(8) The stomach wall contracts and relaxes, which continues mechanical digestion.

(9) Food travels along the oesophagus by peristaltic waves.

(10) Bile is added to the chyme delivered from the gall bladder via the common bile duct.

(11) The pyloric sphincter controls the release of chyme into the small intestine. There it is moved along by peristalsis.

(12) The remnants of the food move into the large intestine where water, electrolytes and water-soluble vitamins are absorbed through the colonic wall.

(13) Food is chewed (masticated) and manipulated into a manageable size by the teeth and tongue. (NB Dogs and cats do not grind their food like herbivores and humans.)

(14) Microbes in the large intestine break down the food remnants and faecal matter is formed.

(15) Food is mixed with saliva and moulded into a bolus by the tongue.

(16) Pancreatic juice is added to the chyme delivered via two pancreatic ducts.

(17) Food is mixed with mucus and gastric juice produced by the glands in the stomach wall. Hydrochloric acid in gastric juice produces an acidic environment.

Activity

Exercise 9.9 Fill in the following chart to show how long it takes food to reach each of the following organs from the oral cavity.

Stomach	(1)
Small intestine	(2)
Rectum	(3)

Activity

Prepare a five-minute presentation entitled 'What happens to a piece of food when an animal eats it?' Your audience could be friends, family or fellow students. When you have finished, invite questions from the floor!

Digestive enzymes

Key Points:

1. An enzyme is a type of protein that causes a biochemical reaction.
2. There are several digestive juices, each containing one or more digestive enzymes.
3. Some digestive juices are secreted from the GI wall; others enter the tract via ducts, e.g. pancreatic juice and bile.

Tip *Enzymes often end with the suffix –ase.*

The breakdown of nutrients

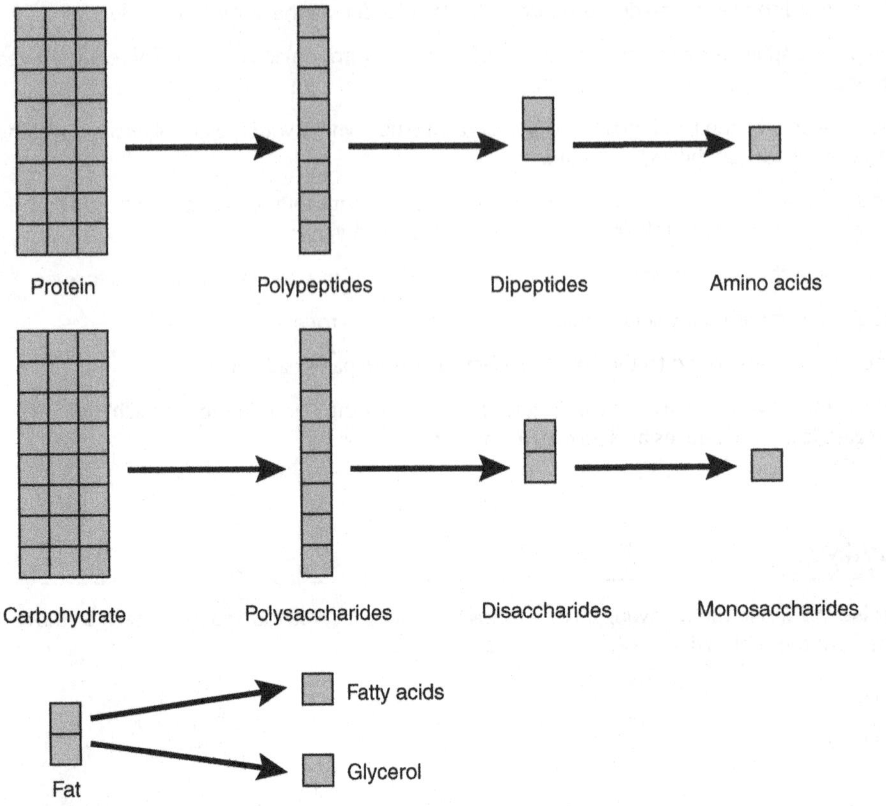

Figure 9.6 The breakdown of nutrients.

Activity

Photocopy (or copy) this chart onto a large sheet of paper and cut out each individual box. Shuffle the boxes and piece the chart back together. This 'jigsaw puzzle' can be used several times to help you learn!

Table 9.2 Contents and functions of the digestive secretions

Secretion	Source	Site of action	Enzymes	Acts on	To produce	Other constituents
Saliva	Salivary glands	Mouth	None	Food	Lubrication	Water, mucus
Gastric juice	Stomach wall	Stomach	Pepsin* Lipase	Protein Fat	Polypeptides Early fat breakdown	Hydrochloric acid
Bile	Liver	Duodenum	Bile salts	Fat	Emulsified fat droplets	Bile pigments, bicarbonate
Pancreatic juice	Pancreas	Duodenum	Trypsin* Peptidases* Amylase Lipase*	Polypeptides Dipeptides Carbohydrate Fat droplets	Dipeptides Amino acids Polysaccharides Fatty acids, glycerol	Bicarbonate
Intestinal juice	Small intestinal wall	Small intestine	Peptidases* Disaccharidases**	Dipeptides Disaccharides	Amino acids Monosaccharides	Mucus, bicarbonate

* Peptidases are a group of enzymes that digest proteins. Examples of peptidases are:
- pepsin (turns proteins into polypeptides and dipeptides)
- trypsin (turns polypeptides into dipeptides and amino acids).

** Disaccharidases are a group of enzymes that digest disaccharides. Examples of disaccharides are:
- lactase (turns lactose, found in milk, into galactose and glucose)
- maltase (turns maltose into glucose)
- sucrase (turns sucrose into fructose and glucose).

Mnemonic

To remember the digestive enzymes:

Perfect **p**ractice **t**akes **c**ommitment **a**nd **d**edication **f**rom **L**isa

Proteins:
Pepsin
Trypsin
Carbohydrates:
Amylase
Disaccharidases
Fats:
Lipase

Faeces and defecation

Key Points:

1. Defecation is a reflex action that is prevented or assisted by the voluntary action of the external anal sphincter.
2. During defecation, faeces move down the anal canal from the rectum and are passed out of the anus.
3. It is normal for dogs and cats to pass faeces two to three times daily.
4. Each time faeces are passed, a small amount of anal sac secretion is squeezed onto the faecal matter; this has a scenting function for territorial marking.

Study

Exercise 9.10 Normal faeces are brown due the presence of bile pigments, a product of erythrocyte breakdown in the liver that has reached the faecal matter via bile. However, both the colour and consistency of faeces can vary. Give reasons for the following:

Pale faeces
Fatty faeces (steatorrhoea)
Mucoid faeces
Black faeces
Dry faeces
Liquid faeces (diarrhoea)

Constituents of faeces

- water
- undigested or partially digested food
- indigestible food, e.g. fibre
- waste products, e.g. bile pigments
- microbes from the large intestine
- mucus from the intestinal wall
- epithelial cells from the wall of the GI tract
- hair, bone or other foreign bodies, e.g. tin foil
- parasites.

General revision

Multiple choice questions

Exercise 9.11

1. The bones that make up the hard palate are the:
   a. palatine, maxilla and incisive bones
   b. maxilla, incisive and lacrimal bones
   c. mandible, incisive and palatine bones
   d. palatine, mandible and lacrimal bones.
2. The bones that have alveolar cavities are the:
   a. maxillae, incisive and lacrimal bones
   b. mandibles and temporal bones
   c. maxillae and parietal bones
   d. mandibles, maxillae and incisive bones.
3. The dental arch is the name for:
   a. the curve on the crown of teeth
   b. all teeth on either jaw, i.e. upper and lower
   c. the curve of the root of teeth
   d. all teeth on either side, i.e. left and right.
4. A cusp is:
   a. another term for a deciduous tooth
   b. one of the cone-shaped prominences on a tooth
   c. another term for a permanent tooth
   d. one of the grooves between the roots of double-rooted teeth.
5. There are no flat surfaces on the teeth of dogs and cats because:
   a. their jaw shape does not allow it
   b. they would be too vulnerable to damage
   c. they do not grind their food
   d. the flat teeth are shed early in life.

6. Ptyalin is:
   a. mucus produced by the mucous membrane of the oral cavity
   b. salivary amylase found in some animals not including dogs and cats
   c. the paste-like matter that leaves the stomach during digestion
   d. the pigment that gives faecal matter its brown colour.
7. The function of hydrochloric acid in the stomach is to:
   a. digest food
   b. create the environment necessary for pepsin production
   c. prevent reflux
   d. create the environment necessary for bile production.
8. Stomach capacity is:
   a. 0.5–8 ml depending on the animal's size
   b. 50–80 ml depending on the animal's size
   c. 0.5–8 l depending on the animal's size
   d. 50–80 l depending on the animal's size.
9. The environment of the small intestine is:
   a. extremely acidic
   b. slightly acidic
   c. extremely alkaline
   d. slightly alkaline.
10. Villi are most numerous in the:
    a. duodenum
    b. jejunum
    c. ileum
    d. colon.
11. Borborygmi are:
    a. non-ruminant herbivores
    b. audible gurgling noises made by the small intestine
    c. muscular contractions of the small intestine
    d. omnivorous animals.
12. Bile is produced in the:
    a. stomach
    b. liver
    c. pancreas
    d. gall bladder.
13. Bile pigment is a product of:
    a. urea formation
    b. poison metabolism
    c. iron storage
    d. erythrocyte breakdown.
14. The liver stores glucose in the form of:
    a. fatty acids
    b. glucagon
    c. glycogen
    d. amino acids.

15. The falciform ligament attaches the liver to the:
    a. diaphragm
    b. stomach
    c. spleen
    d. duodenum.
16. Trypsin acts on:
    a. proteins
    b. fats
    c. carbohydrates
    d. minerals.
17. The disaccharide lactose is found mainly in:
    a. meat
    b. cereal
    c. milk
    d. sugar beet.
18. Proteins are broken down into:
    a. fatty acids
    b. glucose
    c. amino acids
    d. glycerol.
19. Carbohydrates are otherwise known as:
    a. starch, sugars and fibre
    b. oil
    c. the water-soluble vitamins
    d. ash.
20. Approximately how many hours after eating will a dog pass the faeces formed from the meal?
    a. 1–2
    b. 3–5
    c. 12–24
    d. 48–72.

Tip: *Why not get together with fellow students and write some more questions for each other?*

Word chart

Exercise 9.12

1	D
2	I
3	G
4	E
5	S
6	T
7	I
8	O
9	N
10	I
11	N
12	D
13	O
14	G
15	S
16	A
17	N
18	D
19	C
20	A
21	T
22	S

Clues

1. The correct term for the body of the stomach.
2. A small single-rooted tooth designed to hold prey.
3. The prefix pertaining to the stomach.
4. The prefix pertaining to the intestine.
5. The enzyme that breaks down fat.
6. Fat is broken down into glycerol and these substances.
7. Carbohydrates consisting of two monosaccharides.
8. The part of the oesophagus that enters the stomach.
9. The first section of the small intestine.
10. The final section of the small intestine.
11. The last upper premolar.
12. The sphincter that opens to allow food to enter.
13. The active process of releasing stomach contents from the mouth.
14. Difficulty eating or swallowing.
15. The type of muscle in the smooth intestinal wall.

16. The lateral surfaces of the pharynx.
17. These lymphoid structures lie in fossae.
18. A part of the colon meaning 'going down'.
19. The sphincter controlling release of chyme into the duodenum.
20. The main type of microbe found in the large intestine.
21. The __________ of Lieberkühn
22. The correct term for a lump or mass of food.

Crossword

Exercise 9.13

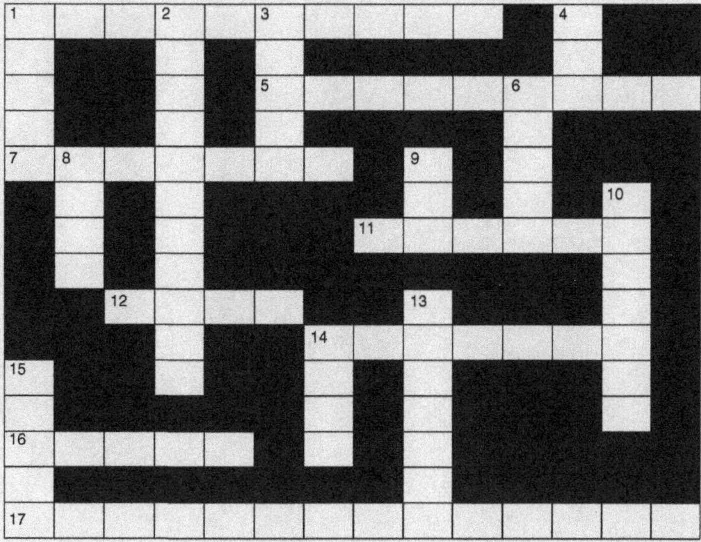

Across	Down
1. Intestinal rumbling noises.	1. A lump or mass of food.
5. Cardiac, pyloric and anal are all one of these.	2. The substance that alters the pH of the environment in the small intestine.
7. When digested this produces fructose and glucose.	3. As something becomes more alkaline, the pH does this.
11. The blind-ending sac in the large intestine.	4. Lay term for the GI tract.
12. Bile acts on these nutrients.	6. A condition caused by violent peristalsis in the intestine which results in severe abdominal pain.

14. Salivary amylase not found in dogs or cats.	8. Formed from ammonia in the liver.
16. The part of the small intestine adjacent to the large intestine.	9. Acronym for the group of substances that includes linoleic acid.
17. A function of the liver.	10. The highly toxic product of fat metabolism.
	13. The most caudal region of the stomach.
	14. Craving for abnormal foodstuffs.
	15. Herbivores' teeth do this but not dogs' and cats'.

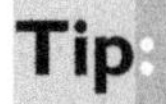

Spend some time looking at radiographs of the GI tract, particularly barium studies. This will help you to learn anatomical positions and transit times.

CHAPTER 10

The urinary system

LEARNING Objectives

This chapter will help you to revise the following:

- facts and functions of the urinary system
- the gross anatomy of the kidney
- the renal nephron
- selective reabsorption
- other functions of the kidney
- the urinary bladder and associated structures
- urine production and micturition.

There is a general revision section at the end of the chapter.

Facts and functions of the urinary system

1. The prefix denoting the urinary system or urine is *urin–*.
2. The prefix denoting the kidney is *nephr–*.
3. The word renal means 'relating to the kidney'.
4. The urinary system has four main components:
   a. the kidneys
   b. the ureters
   c. the urinary bladder
   d. the urethra.
5. The functions of the urinary system are:
   a. the excretion of metabolic wastes and the regulation of the extracellular fluid by urine production
   b. the storage of urine
   c. conversion of vitamin D into its active form
   d. production of the enzyme renin
   e. production of erythropoietin factor.
6. All of these occur in the kidneys except for the storage of urine, which is a function of the urinary bladder.

The gross anatomy of the kidney

Key Points:

1. There are two red–brown bean-shaped kidneys in the dorsal midlumbar region.
2. The right kidney is slightly more cranial than the left.
3. Each kidney is suspended from the dorsal abdominal wall and enveloped in peritoneum; as they do not actually lie inside the peritoneal cavity itself, they are termed *retroperitoneal*.
4. The kidneys are supplied by the renal artery and drained by the renal vein.
5. Each kidney is made up of thousands of individually functioning units called nephrons held together by connective tissue.

Link the words

Exercise 10.1 Match the description in the left-hand column to the correct definition in the right-hand column by drawing a line to link them.

(1)The cup-shaped subdivisions of the ureter within the kidney	(2)Renal cortex
(3)The fibrous connective tissue outer membrane of the kidney, which is protective	(4)Renal hilus
(5)The collecting ducts empty into this area	(6)Renal crest
(7)The outer layer of the kidney where the renal corpuscles are found	(8)Renal medulla
(9)The cone-shaped masses that form the renal medulla	(10)Ureter
(11)The blood vessel that arises directly from the aorta and supplies the kidney	(12)Calyces
(13)The inner region of the kidney where the loops of Henle are found	(14)Renal pelvis
(15)The 'dent' in the kidney where the ureter and blood supply is attached	(16)Renal pyramids
(17)The duct that transports urine from the renal pelvis to the urinary bladder	(18)Renal artery
(19)The area where the collecting ducts merge	(20)Renal capsule

Activity

Exercise 10.2 Below is a diagram of the kidney. From the selection add the correct labels to the diagram.

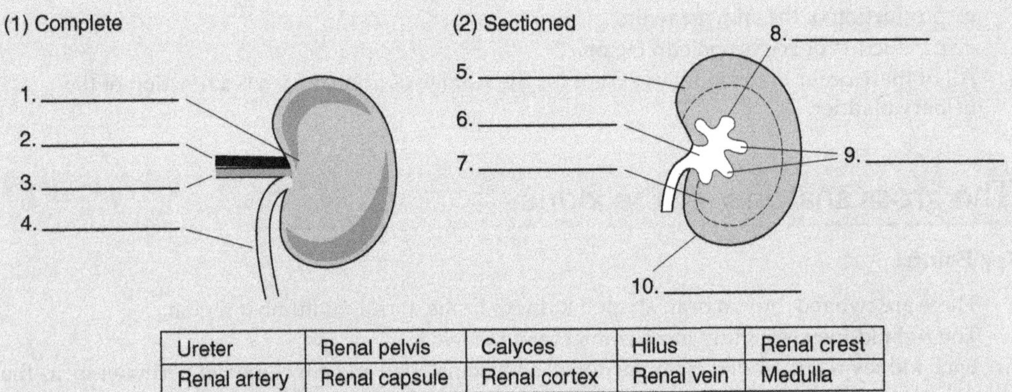

Ureter	Renal pelvis	Calyces	Hilus	Renal crest
Renal artery	Renal capsule	Renal cortex	Renal vein	Medulla

Figure 10.1 Diagram of a kidney.
(Adapted with kind permission from Bowden & Masters 2001.)

The renal nephron

Key Points:

1. The nephron is the functional unit of the kidney.
2. There are around 400,000 nephrons in each canine kidney and around 200,000 nephrons in each feline kidney.
3. Each nephron allows the filtration of blood as it passes through a knot of capillaries called the glomerulus.
4. This filtrate (called glomerular filtrate or ultrafiltrate of plasma) enters the nephron at the Bowman's capsule and moves through the nephron.
5. As the filtrate moves through the nephron, most of it is reabsorbed back into the bloodstream; what remains enters the collecting ducts as urine.
6. Only 0.5–15% of glomerular filtrate ends up as urine; the rest is reabsorbed.
7. Each nephron has remarkable powers of compensation and can filter increasing amounts of blood if other nephrons begin to fail; this is why an animal can still appear clinically normal with only 25% of its nephrons functioning.

Activity

Exercise 10.3 Below is a diagram of the nephron. From the selection add the correct labels.

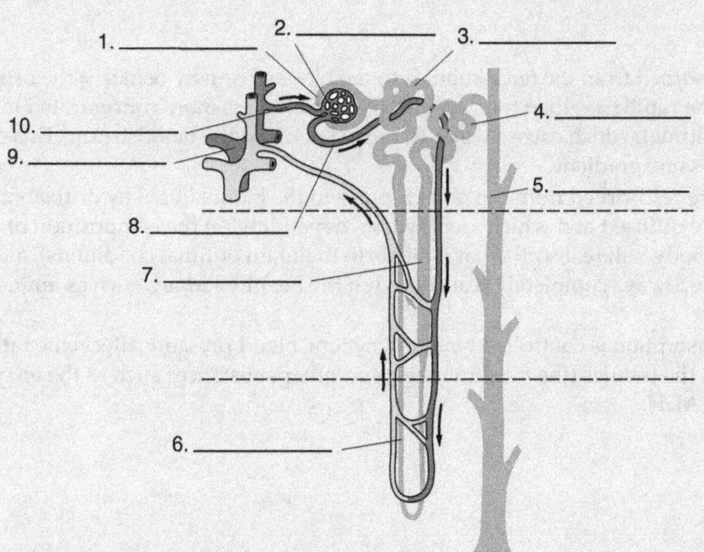

Efferent arteriole	Afferent arteriole	Collecting duct	Glomerulus
Proximal convoluted tubule	Bowman's (glomerular) capsule	Descending loop of Henle	Distal convoluted tubule
Ascending loop of Henle	Renal artery		

Figure 10.2 Diagram of a nephron.
(Reproduced with kind permission from CAW et al 2005.)

Fill in the gaps

Exercise 10.4 Complete the paragraph on the function of the nephron by filling in the gaps using the correct words from the selection below.

- Bowman's
- selective
- proteins
- ECF
- collecting
- glomerulus
- urea
- ultrafiltrate

At the (1)______________, fluid from the bloodstream is filtered through the blood vessel wall and into the (2)______________ capsule. This fluid is called (3)______________ of plasma (or glomerular filtrate). It is very similar to blood plasma except that it does not contain blood cells or the larger plasma (4)______________. The filtrate then moves along the nephron. As it progresses, certain of its constituents are taken back into the bloodstream via the capillaries surrounding the nephron. This is called (5)______________ reabsorption. Only the constituents necessary to the body are reabsorbed such as glucose, amino acids and sufficient of others to maintain optimal conditions in the (6)______________, such as sodium and water. Metabolic waste products, such as (7)______________ and excess amounts of water, sodium, etc., remain in the nephron and pass into the (8)______________ ducts where they move down the ureter into the bladder as urine.

Selective reabsorption

Key Points:

1. Water is reabsorbed from the renal tubules to the bloodstream by osmosis; the osmotic pressure is higher in the capillaries than the nephron (i.e. the blood is more concentrated than the glomerular filtrate), which causes water to move back into the bloodstream. This difference is called the pressure gradient.
2. Substances are reabsorbed from the renal tubules to the bloodstream by diffusion; which substances are diffused and which aren't varies depending on the composition of the ECF at the time (i.e. the body will reabsorb what it needs to maintain optimal conditions), although some substances are always completely reabsorbed in the healthy kidney, such as amino acids and glucose.
3. Selective reabsorption is controlled by many factors; blood pressure affects the rate at which filtrate enters the tubules (the filtration rate) and other substances such as the enzyme renin and the hormone ADH.

Activity

Urea is removed from the body via the kidney. It is common to measure blood urea levels when checking renal function but do you know where urea comes from? Write a paragraph describing the path of urea from its production to its excretion.

Other functions of the kidney

Key Points:

1. The kidney converts fat-soluble vitamin D into active water-soluble vitamin D.
2. The production of the enzyme renin is carried out by the kidney in response to a fall in blood pressure. Renin causes the formation of a substance called angiotensin, which increases blood pressure.
3. Erythropoietin factor, which converts a plasma protein into erythropoietin, is produced in response to a poor oxygen supply to the kidney.

The urinary bladder and associated structures

Key Points:

1. The ureters, bladder and urethra are all lined with transitional epithelium and have smooth muscle in their walls.
2. The two ureters, one from each kidney, enter the bladder on its dorsolateral surface at an oblique angle, creating a flap valve (the ureterovesicular valve) that prevents backflow of urine into the ureters.
3. Urine moves down the ureters by peristalsis.
4. The bladder, positioned on the pelvic floor, extends dorsocranially into the abdominal cavity as it expands to fill with urine.
5. Bladder capacity depends on the size of the animal; a 12.5 kg dog has a bladder capacity of approximately 120 ml.
6. The smooth muscle in the bladder wall is called the *detrusor* muscle.
7. The area of the bladder between the ureters and the bladder neck is called the *vesical trigone.*
8. Urine is prevented from leaking out of the bladder by two sphincter muscles situated at the bladder neck—the internal involuntary sphincter and the external voluntary sphincter.
9. The urethra differs between male and female dogs and cats. In the male it runs between the bladder and the tip of the penis. In the female it runs between the bladder and the junction of the vagina and vestibule.
10. The urethra of the male dog is long and curved whereas in the female dog and cat it is shorter and straight. This, coupled with the presence of the os penis, increases the likelihood of urethral obstruction caused by uroliths, which often become lodged caudal to the os penis.

Activity

Exercise 10.5 Below is a diagram of the urinary system. From the selection add the correct labels.

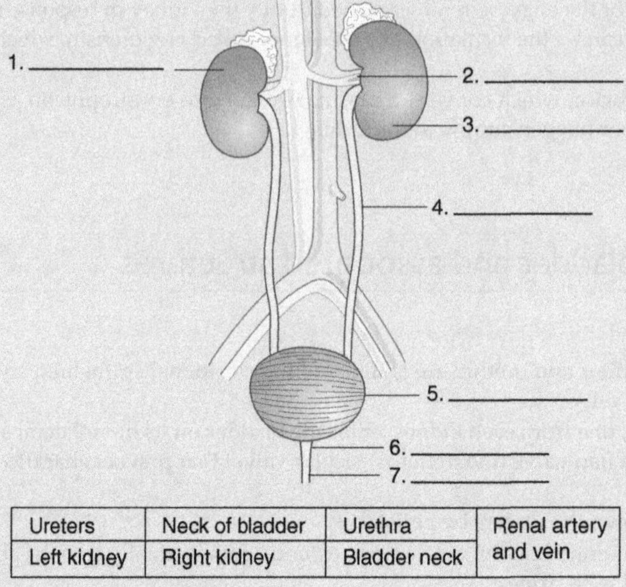

Ureters	Neck of bladder	Urethra	Renal artery and vein
Left kidney	Right kidney	Bladder neck	

Figure 10.3 Diagram of the urinary system.
(Adapted with kind permission from Lane & Cooper 1999.)

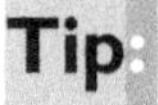

Spend some time looking at abdominal radiographs and identify the bladder. When you get the opportunity, palpate the bladder of a dog or cat. It is also useful to assist with the catheter selection and placement of as many animals as possible!

Urine production and micturition

Key Points:

1. Stretch receptors on the bladder wall indicate when the bladder is full.
2. The internal sphincter is relaxed by a spinal reflex action but the external sphincter is controlled by the brain and is, therefore, under the animal's control.
3. There are many factors affecting urine production including blood pressure, hydration status and health of the urinary tract. For this reason, composition and volume of urine varies, although there are normal ranges.

Activity

Exercise 10.6 Complete the chart below by writing in the normal urine ranges.

	Canine urine	Feline urine
Colour	(1)	(2)
Odour	(3)	(4)
Consistency	(5)	(6)
pH	(7)	(8)
Specific gravity	(9)	(10)
Output (ml/kg/hr)	(11)	(12)

Study

Microscopic analysis of urine is commonly carried out in veterinary practice. List as many things you can think of that could be seen in a sample examined under the microscope.

General revision

Multiple choice questions

Exercise 10.7

1. The renal corpuscle is:
   a. the blood vessel that enters at the hilus
   b. the renal cortex and medulla
   c. the glomerulus and Bowman's capsule
   d. the loop of Henle.
2. The enzyme renin is produced by the kidney in response to:
   a. high blood pressure
   b. low vitamin D levels
   c. low blood pressure
   d. high vitamin D levels.
3. The right ureter is longer than the left ureter because:
   a. it enters the bladder more caudally than the left
   b. it has a slightly smaller diameter than the left
   c. the right kidney produces more urine than the left
   d. the right kidney is more cranial than the left.
4. Which of the following is *not* part of glomerular filtrate?
   a. urea
   b. water
   c. erythrocytes
   d. sodium.

5. The outer membrane of the kidney is the:
   a. cortex
   b. capsule
   c. calyx
   d. crest.
6. Normal canine urine has a specific gravity of:
   a. 5.5–6.5
   b. 1.015–1.045
   c. 6.0–7.0
   d. 1.020.
7. Protein detected in urine may be:
   a. normal
   b. evidence of damage to the urinary tract
   c. evidence of damage to the glomerulus
   d. both b) and c).
8. Which of the following animals has the longest urethra?
   a. male cat
   b. female cat
   c. male dog
   d. female dog.
9. Urine moves along the ureter by:
   a. gravity
   b. peristalsis
   c. osmosis
   d. hydropropulsion.
10. Urine is prevented from moving back up the ureters from the bladder by the:
   a. internal and external sphincters
   b. vesical trigone
   c. ureterovesicular valve
   d. detrusor muscle.

Tip: *Why not get together with fellow students and write some more questions for each other?*

Wordsearch

M	I	C	T	U	R	I	T	I	O	N
P	H	R	B	R	K	M	Z	R	S	E
U	S	E	L	E	C	T	I	V	E	P
L	F	S	N	T	E	B	D	I	L	H
Y	M	T	I	E	W	R	J	T	I	R
N	M	E	N	R	Q	O	E	A	V	I
E	B	Z	E	U	D	S	I	M	E	T
P	T	U	R	E	A	B	S	I	L	I
H	N	T	W	S	C	A	D	N	U	S
R	I	O	P	C	U	E	X	D	B	T
O	G	L	O	M	E	R	U	L	U	S
N	R	U	L	P	H	C	R	U	T	R

Exercise 10.8

- crest
- glomerulus
- reabsorb
- renin
- urea
- selective
- ureter
- nephron
- nephritis
- micturition
- tubule
- vitamin D

Tip: *Have you seen a word you don't understand? Don't ignore it—look it up!*

CHAPTER 11

The reproductive system

LEARNING Objectives

This chapter will help you to revise the following:

- facts and functions of the male reproductive system
- the scrotum, testicles and epididymis
- the spermatic cord and urethra
- the prepuce and penis
- the prostate and bulbo-urethral glands
- facts and functions of the female reproductive system
- the ovary
- the oviduct
- the uterus and cervix
- the vagina and vestibule
- the vulva and clitoris
- the oestrus cycle
- ovulation.

See Chapter 12, 'The Skin and Hair', for information on the mammary glands.

There is a general revision section at the end of this chapter.

THE MALE REPRODUCTIVE SYSTEM

Facts and functions of the male reproductive system

1. The male reproductive system comprises:
   a. the testicles
   b. the epididymis
   c. the scrotum
   d. the spermatic cord
   e. the urethra (shared with the urinary system)
   f. the penis
   g. the prepuce
   h. the prostate gland
   i. the bulbo-urethral glands.
2. The functions of the male reproductive system are:
   a. to produce the male gamete, the spermatozoon (sperm) and seminal fluid
   b. to facilitate mating.
3. The anatomy of the reproductive tracts of male dogs and cats varies quite considerably.
4. The prefix denoting the testes is *orchi–*.
5. The prefix denoting sperm or organs associated with sperm is *spermat–*.

The scrotum, testicles and epididymis

Key Points:

1. The scrotum is a skin-covered sac situated between the hind legs of the dog and between the anus and the prepuce in the cat.
2. The scrotum is situated outside the abdominal cavity as the optimal temperature for spermatogenesis is slightly below normal body temperature.

3. There are two testicles or testes (singular, testicle or testis) lying alongside one another inside the scrotum, separated by a testicular septum. They are fairly mobile in the dog but less so in the cat.
4. It is usual in the dog for the left testicle to be positioned slightly more caudal than the right testicle.
5. Each testicle is supplied by a testicular artery, which branches directly from the aorta. As the blood moves towards the testicle, it is cooled by blood leaving the testicle. This occurs due to the testicular vein forming a convoluted mesh around the testicular artery; this is called the pampiniform plexus.
6. The functions of the testicles are:
   a. the production of the male gamete (the sperm) by the spermatogonia
   b. the production of the hormone oestrogen and nutritive fluid for the sperm by the Sertoli cells
   c. the production of the hormone testosterone by the Leydig cells.
7. The epididymis lies alongside each testicle in the scrotum. Sperm is carried to the epididymis via the efferent ducts, where it is stored.

Link the words

Exercise 11.1 Match the description in the left-hand column to the correct description in the right-hand column by drawing a line to link them.

(1)Seminiferous tubules	(2)Connective tissue divisions in the testicle
(3)Epididymis	(4)The structure containing the deferent duct
(5)Septa	(6)The site of sperm production
(7)Spermatic cord	(8)A double layer of peritoneum, which lines the testicles
(9)Efferent tubules	(10)The site of sperm storage
(11)Tunica vaginalis	(12)The ducts carrying sperm from the testicle to the epididymis

Activity

Exercise 11.2 Below is a diagram of a testicle. From the selection, add the correct labels.

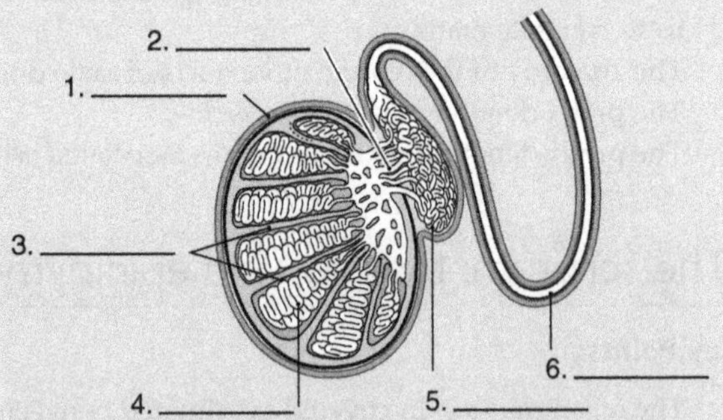

Seminiferous tubules	Septa	Efferent tubules
Epididymis	Spermatic cord	Tunica vaginalis

Figure 11.1 Diagram of a testicle.
(Adapted with kind permission from Reece 1997.)

Look it up

Exercise 11.3 In the embryo, the testicles develop intra-abdominally and are attached to the scrotum by the fibrous gubernaculum, which pulls them through the inguinal canal into the scrotum. In the spaces provided below, write the age you would expect the testicles to have fully descended.

Dog

Cat

Spermatogenesis and sperm structure

A spermatogonium (stem or germ cell) in the seminiferous tubules divides firstly by mitosis then by meiosis to produce immature sperm (spermatids). These mature into sperm in the tubules.

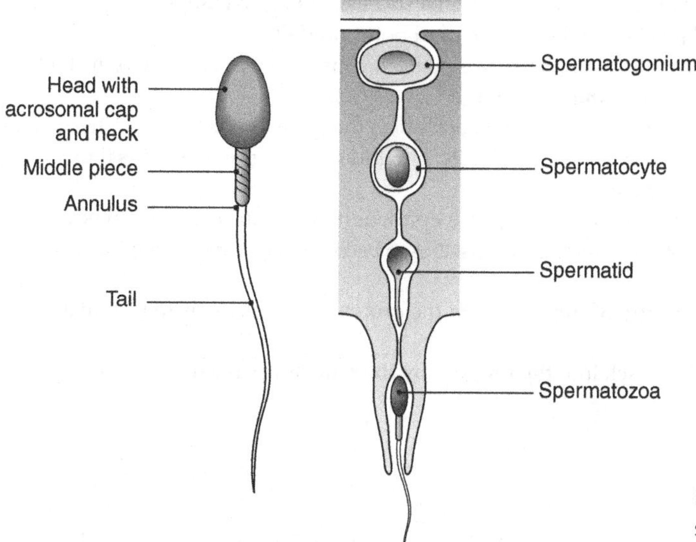

Figure 11.2 Diagram of spermatogenesis and sperm structure. (Adapted with kind permission from Reece 1997.)

The spermatic cord and urethra

Key Points:

1. The spermatic cord runs from the epididymis to the urethra.
2. The spermatic cord comprises the:
   a. deferent duct (*vas deferens*), which is the tube that carries sperm
   b. testicular artery and vein
   c. nerve supply
   d. lymphatic supply
   e. cremaster muscle, which can alter the proximity of the testicles in relation to the body; this is a temperature control mechanism.
3. All components of the spermatic cord are contained within the tunica vaginalis.
4. The spermatic cord moves through the inguinal canal and into the abdominal cavity.

5. The deferent duct opens out into the urethra, which is shared with the urinary tract.
6. The urethra varies in length and shape between dogs and cats:
   a. in the dog, it is long and curved
   b. in the cat, it is short and straight.

Study

It is common practice to castrate dogs and cats but some species are vasectomized. Find out the difference between castration and vasectomy.

The prepuce and penis

Key Points:

1. The prepuce and penis are situated in different regions in dogs and cats:
   a. in the dog they are situated on the ventral abdominal surface and point cranially
   b. in the cat they are situated just below the testicles and point caudally.
2. The prepuce (or sheath) houses the distal part of the penis. Its outer surface is covered in skin but its inner surface is lined with mucous membrane.
3. The prepuce protects the penis and is only drawn back when the penis is erect.
4. The penis comprises mainly erectile tissue, which fills with blood during sexual arousal to distend the penis and allow mating to occur.
5. In the dog, the surface of the penis is smooth mucous epithelium but in the cat it is barbed.
6. In dogs and some cats an area of the erectile tissue ossifies to become a U-shaped bone (the os penis).
7. The urethra runs through the centre of the penis and the groove of the os penis to terminate at its tip.
8. After mating, the penis is pulled back into the prepuce by the retractor penis muscle.

Activity

Exercise 11.4 Below is a diagram of the penis of the dog. From the selection, add the correct labels.

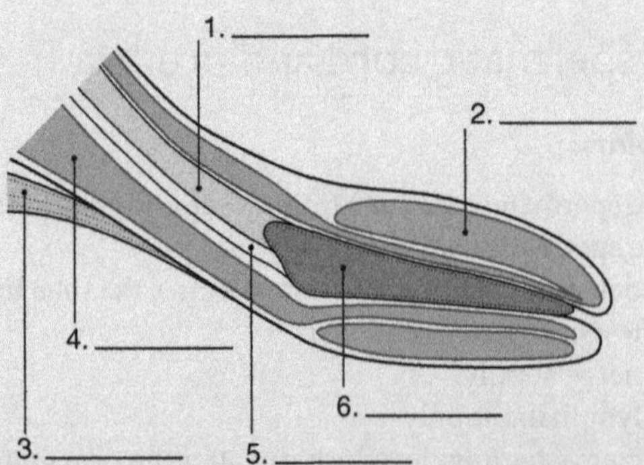

Figure 11.3 Diagram of a penis.
(Adapted with kind permission from Evans 1993.)

Corpus cavernosum	Corpus spongiosum	Bulbus glandis
Retractor penis	Os penis	Urethra

The mechanism of erection

1. Sexual arousal causes the arteries supplying the penis to dilate, increasing blood flow.
2. Drainage of the blood is slowed by inhibition of the venous supply caused by contraction of muscles surrounding the penis.
3. Blood enters the large spaces in the erectile tissue causing it to distend.
4. After ejaculation, the surrounding muscles relax to allow venous drainage to occur and the arteries reduce in size.

The prostate gland and the bulbo-urethral glands

Key Points:

1. The prostate and bulbo-urethral glands produce seminal fluid, which makes up the volume of the ejaculate.
2. This fluid contains nutrients to support the sperm once they have left the male reproductive tract.
3. The prostate is situated at the junction of the deferent duct and urethra. It completely surrounds the urethra.
4. The prostate is oval shaped with a sulcus (groove) running down its centre.
5. The paired bulbo-urethral glands are situated further down the urethra in the cat but are not present in the dog.
6. The secretion from both glands is delivered into the urethra via ducts.

Study

The prostate gland varies in size according to the breed, size and age of the animal. However, abnormal enlargement of the prostate is very common in older dogs. What symptoms do these animals show and what is the common treatment for this problem?

THE FEMALE REPRODUCTIVE SYSTEM

Facts and functions of the female reproductive system

1. The functions of the female reproductive tract are:
   a. to produce the ova (singular, ovum), the female gamete
   b. to facilitate mating
   c. to provide the correct environment for fertilization and development of the embryo
   d. to allow parturition to occur at the correct time
   e. to enable feeding of the neonate by lactation.
2. The prefixes denoting ova are *ovi–* or *oo–*.
3. The prefix denoting the uterus is *metr–*.

The ovary

Key Points:

1. The ovary is the female gonad, producing the female gamete (the ovum).
2. There are two ovaries situated in the dorsal abdominal cavity, just caudal to the kidneys and suspended from the dorsal abdominal wall by a fold of peritoneum (the mesovarium). This narrows into a ligament, the ovarian (suspensory) ligament, which then opens out completely enveloping the ovary, forming a bursa.

3. The ovary is a raspberry-like structure in appearance but this varies depending on the animal's age, pregnancy status and stage of cycle.
4. The ovary is supplied by the ovarian artery, which branches directly from the aorta.
5. The ovary is made from connective tissue and interspersed with ovarian follicles at various stages of development.
6. An ovarian follicle is a secretory sac; each contains an immature ovum, which will not mature until influenced hormonally.
7. An animal is born with its full complement of immature ova and follicles. A small number mature during each oestrus cycle.
8. In addition to oocyte maturation and release, the ovary also produces oestrogen. (See 'Ovulation' below and Ch. 6, 'The Endocrine System', for more information.)

Activity

Exercise 11.5 Below is a diagram of an ovary. From the selection add the correct labels.

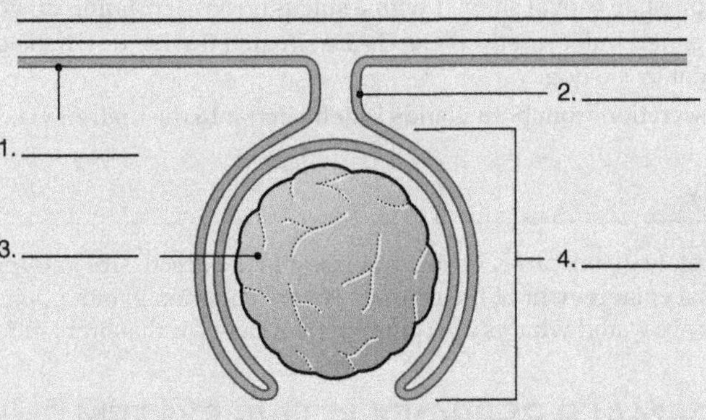

Ovarian (suspensory) ligament	Ovarian bursa
Ovary	Fold of peritoneum becoming mesovarium

Figure 11.4 Diagram of an ovary.

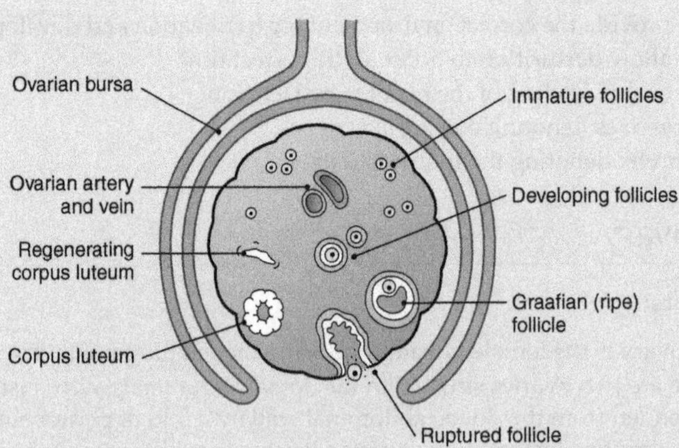

Figure 11.5 The complete microstructure of the ovary.

The oviduct

Key Points:

1. The oviduct is also called the fallopian tube or uterine tube.
2. One oviduct runs from each ovary to the uterus and is suspended from the dorsal abdominal wall by the mesosalpinx.
3. The ovarian end of the oviduct flares out to enclose the ovary; this funnel-shaped area is called the infundibulum.
4. The infundibulum is fringed with finger-like projections called fimbriae, which assist ova to move into the oviduct.
5. The oviduct is lined with ciliated columnar epithelium; the cilia also assist in the movement of ova.
6. The oviduct is the site for fertilization of the ova with the male gamete (the spermatozoon).

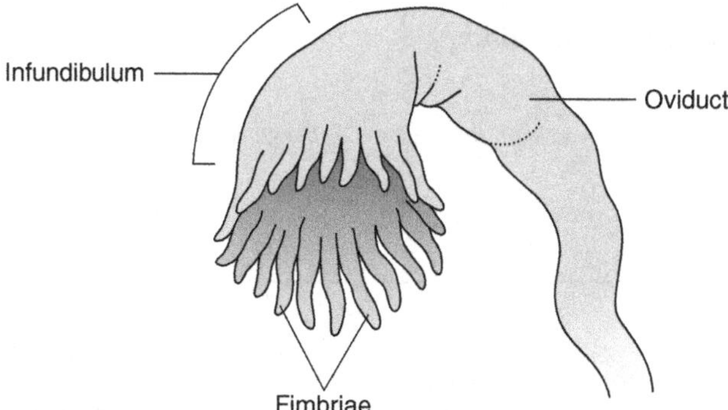

Figure 11.6 Diagram of the oviduct.

The uterus and cervix

Key Points:

1. The function of the uterus is to provide a suitable site for implantation and development of the conceptus and associated membranes.
2. The uterus is Y-shaped in dogs and cats, having long horns and a short body.
3. A non-pregnant uterus lies fairly dorsal in the abdominal cavity, running between the oviducts and the cervix. However, during pregnancy, the weight of the uterus causes it to move more ventrally.
4. The uterus is suspended from the dorsal abdominal cavity by a fold of peritoneum (the mesometrium).
5. The wall of the uterus (myometrium) comprises several layers of smooth muscle.
6. The inner lining of the uterus (endometrium) is highly glandular. Its thickness and composition varies according to the animal's age, pregnancy status and stage of cycle.
7. The cervix is the protective entrance of the uterus and it projects into the vagina. It is a highly muscular sphincter that remains tightly closed except during oestrus, mating and parturition.

Study

Uterine shapes vary between species. Find out the shapes of the horse, cattle and pig uteri. Why do you think they differ?

The vagina and vestibule

Key Points:

1. The vagina and vestibule together make up the genital passage or birth canal.
2. The vagina is situated between the cervix and the vestibule. It terminates at the external urethral orifice. Its stratified squamous mucosal lining is arranged in longitudinal folds and smooth muscle is present in its wall.
3. The lining of the vagina changes in thickness and appearance during various stages of the oestrus cycle under hormonal influence.
4. The vestibule is situated between the vagina and the vulva. It begins at the external urethral orifice. There are no longitudinal folds in its lining.
5. The genital passage has four functions:
   a. passage of sperm
   b. housing the penis during mating
   c. passage of the fetus during parturition
   d. passage of urine exiting from the external urethral orifice.

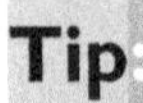

Assisting with the catheterization of a bitch will help you learn the anatomy of the genital passage!

Vulva and clitoris

Key Points:

1. The vulva is the terminal part of the female reproductive tract.
2. At the entrance to the vulva are the vulval labiae (singular, labia) or vulval lips, which may swell at various stages of the oestrus cycle.
3. A small area of erectile tissue, the clitoris, sits at the base of the vulva. It contains sensory nerve endings and very occasionally a bone, the *os clitoridis.*

The oestrus cycle

Key Points:

1. Bitches are seasonally monoestrus, i.e. they only have one oestrus cycle per season and have approximately two breeding seasons per year. Timing of the seasons is affected by many factors, including photoperiod and synchronization between bitches living as a group.
2. Queens are seasonally polyoestrus, i.e. they may have many oestrus cycles per season. The breeding season of the queen runs from February to September and is dictated by photoperiod.
3. The oestrus cycle has four stages:
   a. proestrus; the female is attractive to the male but will not allow mating. The vulval lips are extremely swollen and there is a bloody discharge apparent
   b. oestrus; the female will allow mating, and ovulation occurs. The vulval lips remain swollen but become softer and the discharge becomes straw coloured
   c. metoestrus (or dioestrus); the female is no longer attractive to the male or interested in mating. Vulval swelling and discharge disappear. Mammary development occurs and pseudopregnancy occurs in non-pregnant bitches
   d. anoestrus; a period of quiescence. Clinical signs regress.

OESTRUS

- Approx. 7 days (range 3–21 days)
- Oestrogen dominance in early oestrus
- LH surge causes ovulation
- Progesterone dominance in late oestrus

- Swollen but soft vulva
- Serous straw coloured discharge
- Will stand for male
- Tail deviation

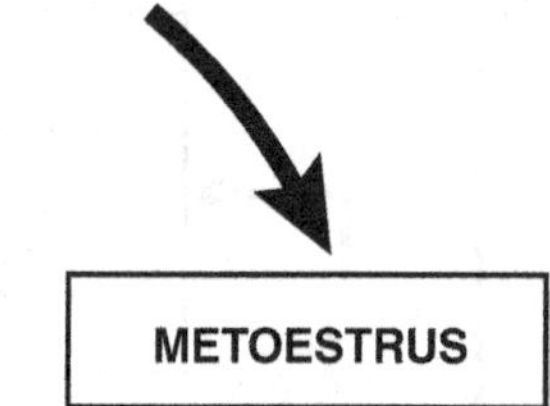

PROESTRUS

- Approx. 9 days (range 2–27 days)
- FSH develops follicles
- LH in late proestrus
- Oestrogen levels increase
- Swollen firm vulva
- Bloody discharge
- Attractive to male but will not stand for male
- Polyuria

METOESTRUS

- Approx. 60 days (range 30–90 days)
- Progesterone levels increase at first
- Progesterone levels decrease later and prolactin is released
- Vulval swelling and discharge slowly diminish
- Pseudopregnancy occurs in late metoestrus

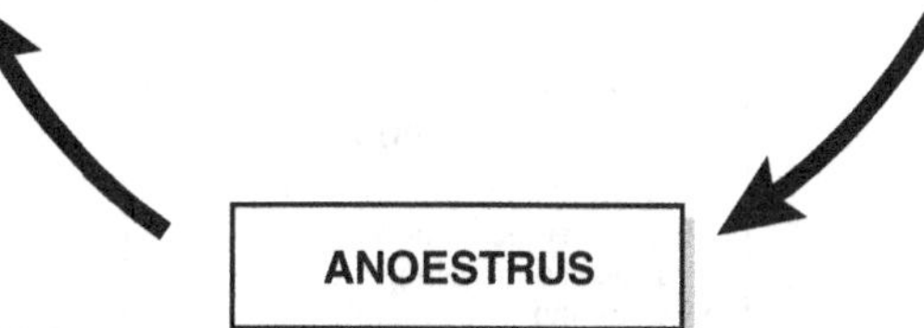

ANOESTRUS

- Approx. 4 months (length dictates frequency of season)
- Hormonal activity stabilizes and there is a period of quiet
- Normal appearance and behaviour

Figure 11.7 Diagram of the oestrus cycle of the bitch.

Look it up

Exercise 11.6 Complete the chart below by filling in information in the correct boxes.

Stage	Approximate length	Hormones involved	Clinical signs
Proestrus	(1)	(2)	(3)
Oestrus	(4)	(5)	(6)
Metoestrus	(7)	(8)	(9)
Anoestrus	(10)	(11)	(12)

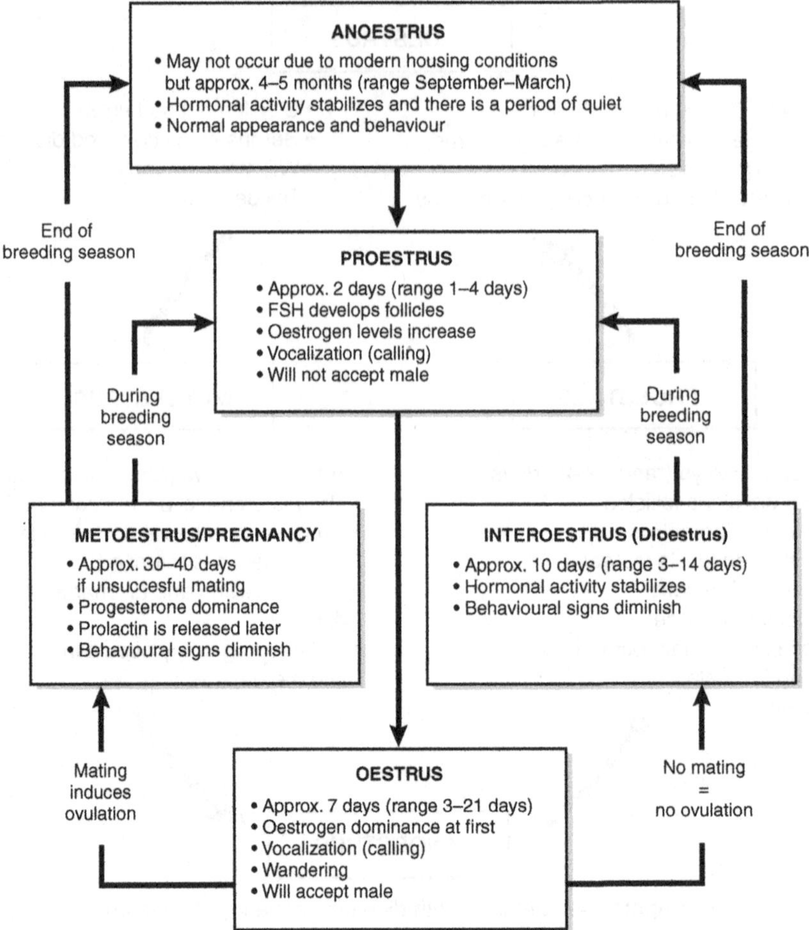

Figure 11.8 Diagram of the oestrus cycle of the queen.

Ovulation

Key Points:

1. Ovulation is the process of an ovum being released from a mature (graafian) follicle and leaving the ovary.
2. Ovulation begins to occur at approximately six months of age and continues throughout the animal's reproductive life.
3. Ovulation occurs at the oestrus stage of the oestrus cycle and is triggered by a surge of luteinizing hormone (LH).
4. Ovulation in the bitch is spontaneous, i.e. no stimulation is needed. However, in the queen, ovulation must be induced by mating.
5. The number of ova released during each cycle varies between species, but in the dog and cat, an average of 5 to 12 in total come from both ovaries.
6. A released ovum survives for 3 or 4 days in the reproductive tract.

Activity

Exercise 11.7 Photocopy (or copy) the ovulation chart below onto a large piece of paper and cut out each individual statement. Then arrange the statements in the order in which they occur.

(1)The same process occurs whether or not the animal is pregnant.

(2)Each corpus luteum continues to develop for approximately 30 days. This is known as the luteal phase.

(3)Some bleeding occurs in the follicles, which then become solid structures and secrete progesterone, the hormone that maintains pregnancy.

(4)A number of immature follicles in the ovary begin to mature under the hormonal influence of follicle-stimulating hormone (FSH) and LH.

(5)The released ova move down the oviduct where fertilization will take place if mating has occurred.

(6)The maturing follicles enlarge and fill with fluid. They begin to move towards the edge of the ovary.

(7)These solid structures are corpora lutea (singular, corpus luteum).

(8)After this each corpus luteum begins to degenerate until it cannot secrete enough progesterone to maintain pregnancy. This occurs at day 63–65 after ovulation and is one of the triggers for parturition.

(9)The fully mature (graafian) follicles protrude from the edge of the ovary and, under the influence of a surge of LH, they rupture to release the ova inside.

General revision

Multiple choice questions – the male reproductive system

Exercise 11.8

1. The fibrous structure that pulls the testicle into the scrotum during development is the:
   a. cremaster muscle
   b. gubernaculum
   c. pampiniform plexus
   d. corpus cavernosum.
2. In the dog, testicles should have descended into the scrotum by:
   a. birth
   b. 5–10 days of age
   c. 30–40 days of age
   d. six months of age.
3. The cells that produce testosterone are:
   a. Leydig cells
   b. germ cells
   c. Sertoli cells
   d. prostate cells.

4. Which of the following structures is not part of the spermatic cord?
   a. deferent duct
   b. testicular artery
   c. urethra
   d. lymphatic vessel.
5. Sperm is stored in the:
   a. seminiferous tubules
   b. epididymis
   c. deferent duct
   d. penis.
6. The prostate gland produces:
   a. seminal fluid
   b. sperm
   c. mucous
   d. muscle fibres.
7. An animal with both testicles retained intra-abdominally is said to be:
   a. bilaterally anorchid
   b. unilaterally monorchid
   c. bilaterally cryptorchid
   d. unilaterally anorchid.
8. The condition in which the penis protrudes from the prepuce and cannot be retracted is called:
   a. prostatitis
   b. dysuria
   c. tenesmus
   d. paraphimosis.

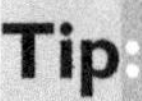
Why not get together with fellow students and write some more questions for each other?

Look it up

Exercise 11.9 Fill in the chart below to describe the differences between the reproductive tracts of male dogs and cats.

	Dogs	**Cats**
Position of testes	(1)	(2)
Hair distribution on scrotum	(3)	(4)
Presence of bulbo-urethral glands	(5)	(6)
Position of the penis and prepuce	(7)	(8)
Presence of os penis	(9)	(10)
Texture of penis surface	(11)	(12)
Length and shape of urethra	(13)	(14)

Activity

Exercise 11.10 Below is a diagram of the male reproductive tract of the dog. From the selection add the correct labels.

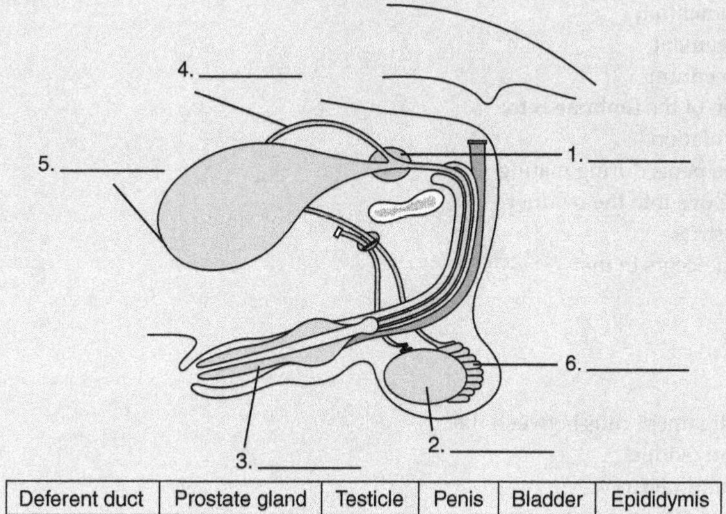

Deferent duct	Prostate gland	Testicle	Penis	Bladder	Epididymis

Figure 11.9 Diagram of the male reproductive tract.
(Reproduced with kind permission from CAW et al 2005.)

Multiple choice questions – the female reproductive system

Exercise 11.11

1. The mesovarium, mesosalpinx and mesometrium make up the:
   a. broad ligament
   b. greater omentum
   c. round ligament
   d. lesser omentum.
2. The function of the fimbriae is to:
   a. cause ovulation
   b. house the penis during mating
   c. draw the ova into the oviduct
   d. cause oestrus.
3. Fertilization occurs in the:
   a. ovary
   b. oviduct
   c. uterus
   d. vagina.
4. The round ligament runs between the:
   a. ovary and oviduct
   b. oviduct and uterus
   c. uterus and inguinal ring
   d. vagina and inguinal ring.
5. The inner lining of the uterus is the:
   a. mesometrium
   b. pyometrium
   c. myometrium
   d. endometrium.
6. The cervix is largely made up of:
   a. connective tissue
   b. epithelial tissue
   c. nervous tissue
   d. muscle tissue.
7. The female homologue of the penis is the:
   a. vagina
   b. clitoris
   c. vulva
   d. uterus.
8. The genital passage comprises the:
   a. ovary, oviduct, uterus and cervix
   b. uterus, cervix and vagina
   c. vagina and vestibule
   d. vestibule.

9. The external urethral orifice is situated between the:
   a. vagina and vestibule
   b. cervix and vagina
   c. vestibule and vulva
   d. vulva and anus.
10. The stages of the oestrus cycle that occur when a bitch is 'in season' are:
    a. proestrus and oestrus
    b. oestrus and metoestrus
    c. metoestrus and anoestrus
    d. anoestrus and proestrus.
11. A straw-coloured discharge occurs during:
    a. proestrus
    b. oestrus
    c. metoestrus
    d. anoestrus.
12. Pseudopregnancy occurs during:
    a. proestrus
    b. oestrus
    c. metoestrus
    d. anoestrus.
13. A mature follicle is called a:
    a. oocyst
    b. graafian follicle
    c. oocyte
    d. Golgi follicle.
14. Induced ovulation occurs:
    a. spontaneously
    b. only when the animal has been mated
    c. only under the influence of drug therapy
    d. rarely in cats and dogs.
15. Seasonally polyoestrus means:
    a. the animal has several oestrus cycles in one breeding season
    b. the animal ovulates several ova in one oestrus cycle
    c. the animal must mate in order to ovulate
    d. the animal has an abnormal number of oestrus cycles per breeding season.

Tip: *Why not get together with fellow students and write some more questions for each other?*

Activity

Exercise 11.12 Below is a diagram of the female reproductive organs. From the selection add the correct labels.

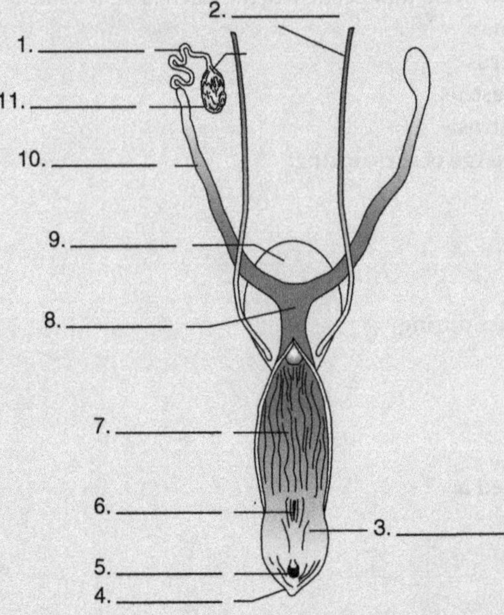

Urinary bladder	Clitoris	Uterine body	External urethral orifice	Uterine horn	Infundibulum
Ovary	Vestibule	Oviduct	Vulva	Vagina	

Figure 11.10 The female reproductive organs.
(Reproduced with kind permission from Colville & Bassert 2002.)

CHAPTER 12

The skin and hair

LEARNING Objectives

This chapter will help you to revise the following:

- facts and functions of the skin and hair
- the structure of the skin
- modified skin and glands
- the formation and structure of hair.

There is a general revision section at the end of the chapter.

Facts and functions of the skin and hair

1. The skin and hair, or integument, completely cover the surface of the body and are continuous with the mucous membrane that lines the orifices of the body.
2. The skin is adapted (modified) in several areas, e.g. the digital pads and the rhinarium.
3. There are several different types of hair distributed in varying quantities throughout the body.
4. The functions of the skin and hair may be grouped into the following categories:
   a. protective
   b. sensory
   c. secretory
   d. productive
   e. thermoregulatory.

Fill in the gaps

Exercise 12.1 Complete the paragraphs by filling in the gaps using the correct words from the selection below.

- pheromones
- pacinian
- sebum
- digital
- vasodilation
- camouflage
- arrector
- vibrissae
- panting
- vasoconstriction
- ergosterol
- sudoriferous
- keratin
- bacteria

Protective functions of the skin

The skin provides protection against physical trauma and weather elements such as sunlight and wind. Invasions of the body by micro-organisms such as (1)__________ are also prevented. To increase protection further, the skin and hair are waterproofed by the oily secretion (2)__________. During a fight or attack, an animal may use its claws; these are made from modified epidermis infiltrated with the tough protein (3)__________. In their wild state, the coats of canines and felines may provide (4)__________ or act as a display or warning signal to other animals. In domestic pets, however, coat colour is now largely dictated by elective breeding, although hair still stands on end as a defence mechanism (hackles in the dog and a spiky tail in the cat).

Sensory functions of the skin

The dermis of the skin contains several different types of nerve ending that detect pressure, pain, heat, cold, etc. These are called sensory receptors. Each sensory receptor is stimulus specific and so does not respond to a different stimulus. Examples of cutaneous sensory receptors are the (5)__________ corpuscles (which detect pressure), Meissner's corpuscles (which detect touch),

Krause's receptors (which detect cold) and Ruffini's corpuscles (which detect heat). 'Whiskers', or (6)______________, are attached to nerve endings that detect movement and play a major sensory role, particularly in the cat.

Secretory functions of the skin

There are two main types of exocrine gland in the dermis. Sebaceous glands produce the oily secretion sebum, which waterproofs the hair. Sebum has a distinctive smell, which acts as an identifying marker. (7)______________, chemical substances used to attract mates, are also found in sebum. (8)______________, or sweat glands, are also present in the dermis. There are two types: eccrine and apocrine. Eccrine glands are only present in the (9)______________ pads of dogs and cats. Their secretion is thought to be useful in increasing traction when running. Apocrine glands are distributed throughout the body. Their secretion mixes with sebum to aid protection of the coat and produce the glossy sheen seen in healthy animals. Neither type of sudoriferous gland is particularly efficient at cooling the body by evaporative heat loss, although some does occur.

Productive function of the skin

Vitamin D precursors (10)______________ and dehydrocholesterol are present in the skin. In the presence of UV light, e.g. sunlight, the precursors become ergocalciferol (vitamin D_2) and cholecalciferol (vitamin D_3).

Thermoregulatory functions of the skin

Fat, present in the hypodermis, insulates the body against cold environmental temperatures. The coat also insulates against cold weather, usually being thicker in winter months. Additionally, erector muscles known as (11)______________ pili contract during cold weather, causing hair to stand up and create pockets of warm air close to the skin (seen as 'goose bumps' in people).

Blood vessels in the dermis constrict (12)(______________) or dilate (13)(______________) in response to decreased or increased temperatures respectively, thus controlling the amount of blood flowing near the body surface where the temperature is cooler.

Evaporative heat loss through sweating does occur but this is not a major cooling method; water evaporation from the mouth and tongue by (14)______________ is far more effective in the dog and cat.

The structure of the skin

Key Points:

1. The skin is made up of three main layers:
   a. the epidermis
   b. the dermis
   c. the hypodermis.
2. The epidermis contains no blood vessels. It is made up of four main layers:
   a. the deepest layer, where epithelial cells divide, is the stratum germinativum
   b. the cells move upwards and flatten, forming the stratum granulosum
   c. the cells move further upwards and begin to lose their nuclei, forming the stratum lucidum
   d. the uppermost layer of the epidermis, the stratum corneum, contains cells that have lost their nuclei and their shape. These cells slowly slough away and are constantly replaced by cells from the stratum lucidum.
3. The tough protein keratin slowly infiltrates the cells to provide extra protection to the epidermis. Keratinization is heavier in certain parts of the body, such as the footpads.
4. The dermis is a dense connective tissue layer, which contains blood vessels, sensory nerve endings, glands and hair follicles. It has round protuberances called dermal papillae on its outermost surface.
5. The hypodermis is, strictly speaking, the layer underneath the skin. It is made up of loose connective tissue and is infiltrated with fat cells. Some deep hair follicles may be found in the hypodermis.

Activity

Exercise 12.2 Below is a diagram depicting a cross-section of the skin. From the selection add the correct labels.

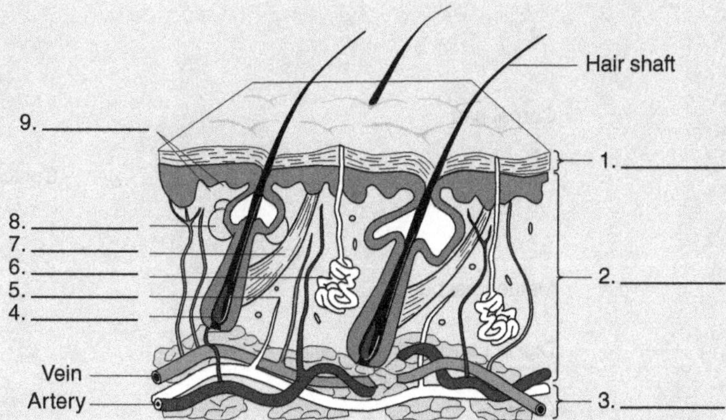

Dermal papillae	Hypodermis	Dermis	Arrector pili muscle	Sudoriferous gland
Sebaceous gland	Hair follicle	Sensory receptor	Epidermis	

Figure 12.1 Diagram of a cross-section through the skin.
(Reproduced with kind permission from Bowden & Masters 2001.)

Modified skin and glands

Key Points:

1. There are several areas of modified skin on the body, including the following:
   a. the rhinarium or nose; there is no stratum granulosum or stratum lucidum, although the epidermal layer is very thick. There is an absence of hair follicles and the area is usually heavily pigmented. The moisture comes mainly from a gland situated just inside the nares. Each individual animal has a unique 'nose print', rather like a person's fingerprint
   b. the digital pads; the stratum corneum is extremely thick and heavily keratinized to provide protection. In the cat the pads are fairly smooth but in the dog they are rough to the touch, being composed of many conical papillae. The hypodermis is infiltrated with fat cells (adipose tissue) to provide a 'shock absorbing' layer
   c. the claws; formed from modified epidermis, the claw projects from the ungual process of the third phalanx of each digit in two sheets, which are joined together by the claw sole. The area where the claw and the ungual process meet is called the coronary border. This sensitive area is hidden by a fold of skin (the claw fold).
2. There are many modified glands on the body, including the following:
   a. the mammary glands; these are modified sudoriferous glands. Dogs and cats have four to six pairs, the males having rudimentary glands

b. the glands of the ear canal; the secretions of the sebaceous and apocrine glands in the auditory canal combine to produce cerumen (earwax)
c. the anal sac glands; circumanal glands and tail glands are all modified sebaceous glands whose main function is scenting or territory marking
d. the meibomian (tarsal) glands of the eyelids whose fatty secretion contributes to tear film.

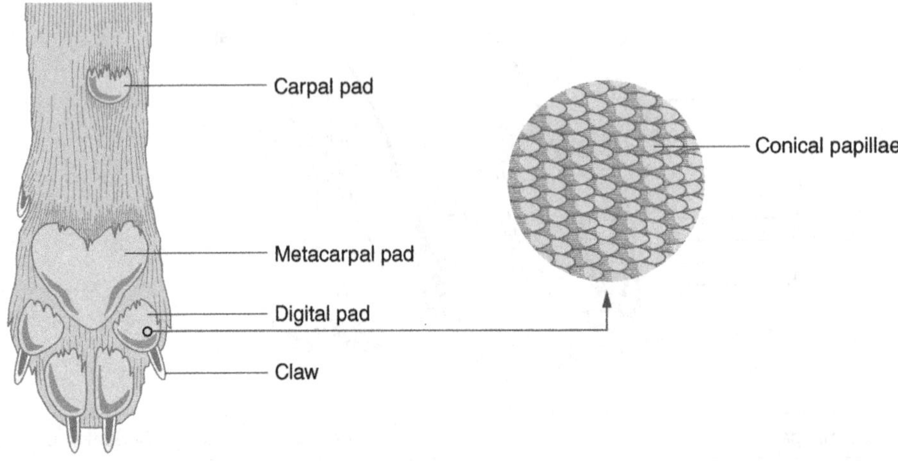

Figure 12.2 Diagram and close-up of the foot pad of a dog.
(Reproduced with kind permission from CAW et al 2005.)

Activity

Exercise 12.3 Below is a diagram depicting a section through a mammary gland. From the selection add the correct labels.

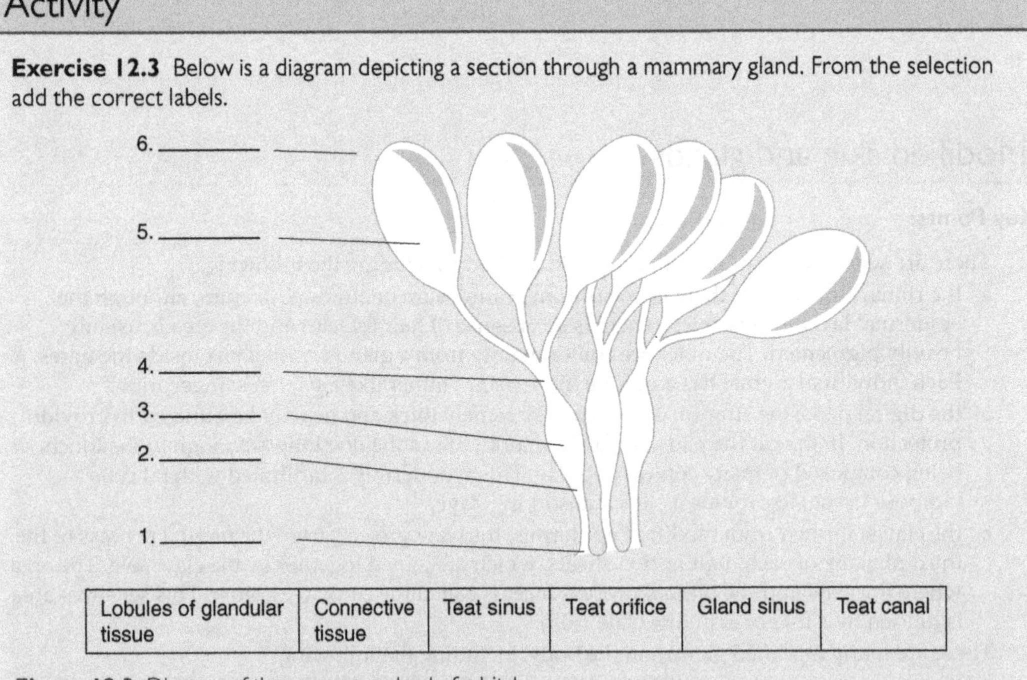

Lobules of glandular tissue	Connective tissue	Teat sinus	Teat orifice	Gland sinus	Teat canal

Figure 12.3 Diagram of the mammary gland of a bitch.
(Reproduced with kind permission from CAW et al 2005.)

Structure and formation of hair

Key Points:

1. There are many different types of hair, although they all have a similar structure:
   a. an outer cuticle
   b. a cortex containing pigmentation
   c. an inner medulla (which is sometimes hollow)
   d. the root of the hair begins with an expanded end (bulb) that grows out of a follicle to form the hair shaft.
2. Associated with each hair follicle are a sebaceous gland and an arrector pili muscle.
3. Hairs are constantly being formed, growing and being shed from the follicles. There are different stages of hair growth:
   a. anagen (the growth stage)
   b. catagen (the shedding stage)
   c. telogen (the resting stage).
4. A new hair forms when epidermis extends downwards covering the dermal papilla beneath it, forming a hair cone. Hair begins to grow from the hair cone through the hair follicle.
5. There are three main types of hair:
   a. guard or topcoat hairs; these are the waterproofing and protective hairs of the coat
   b. wool, lanugo or undercoat hairs; these form the soft insulating layer of the coat
   c. vibrissae, 'whiskers' or sensory hairs; these are specialized hairs attached to nerve endings that detect movement. They are only found in certain areas of the body—upper lip, eyelashes (cilia), eyebrows (superciliary hairs), cheeks and chin (submental hairs). In cats, vibrissae are also found on the carpus.
6. Hair is not evenly distributed throughout the body. Some areas, such as the dorsal cervical area, are very hairy; others are not, such as the ventral abdomen. Some areas have only certain types of hair, such as the scrotum, which does not have wool hairs due to the requirement for lower temperatures required for spermatogenesis.
7. Hair length varies between breeds and individuals. Although it is largely genetically determined, season and temperature also play a part.
8. Growth rate also varies widely, although it does grow more quickly in a colder climate. However, on average, hair grows at approximately 0.04mm per day.
9. Moulting usually occurs during the spring and autumn and lasts approximately five weeks. Some breeds appear to moult more heavily than others; other factors affecting moulting include temperature and photoperiod.

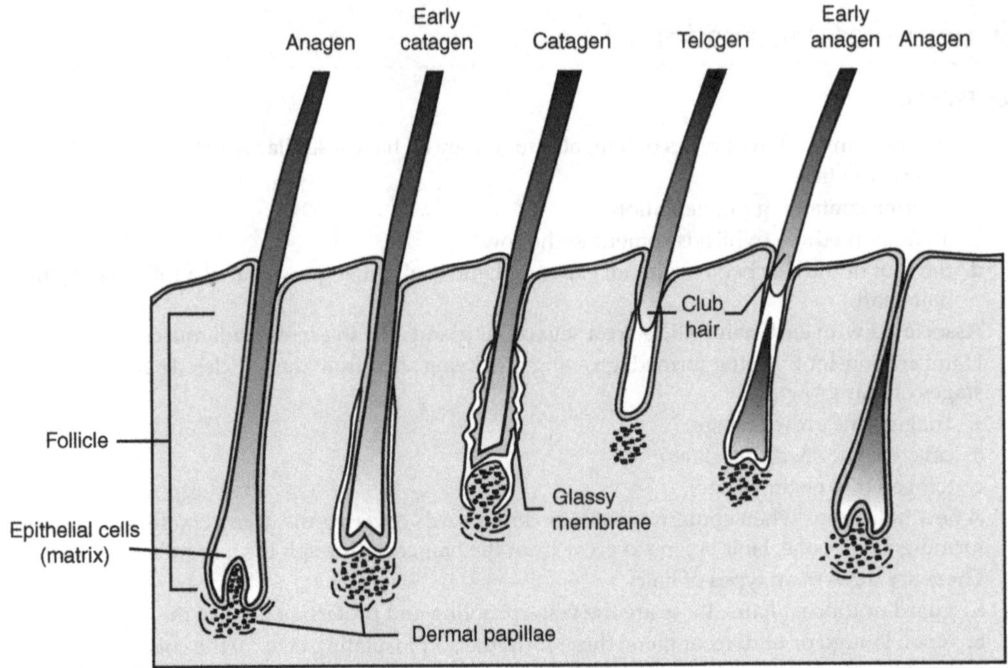

Figure 12.4 The growth cycle of a mammalian hair, showing the three phases (anagen, catagen and telogen). (Reproduced with kind permission from Colville & Bassert 2002.)

Activity

Inspect the coats of several dogs and cats. Try to categorize the coat types by lengths and textures and differentiate between the different hair types.

General revision

Multiple choice questions

Exercise 12.4

1. Integument is another term for:
   a. hairless skin only
   b. the covering of the body including pads, nails and hair
   c. all hairy skin only
   d. the modified areas of skin only, e.g. pads, nails and hair
2. The chemical released from the sebaceous glands to attract the opposite sex is:
   a. sebum
   b. pheromone
   c. sweat
   d. tear film.

3. The sensory receptors that detect touch are:
   a. pacinian corpuscles
   b. Meissner's corpuscles
   c. Krause's end-bulb receptors
   d. Ruffini's corpuscles.
4. Submental vibrissae are found:
   a. on the eyebrows
   b. on the feline carpus
   c. on the cheeks and chin
   d. on the cheeks.
5. Eccrine glands are found:
   a. in the footpads
   b. on the tongue
   c. in the eyelids
   d. on the tail.
6. Arrector pili muscles play a part in:
   a. sensory reception
   b. vitamin D production
   c. movement
   d. thermoregulation.
7. The hypodermis consists of:
   a. dense connective tissue
   b. muscle tissue
   c. loose connective tissue
   d. sebaceous glands.
8. The basement layer of the epidermis is the:
   a. stratum corneum
   b. stratum granulosum
   c. stratum germinativum
   d. stratum lucidum.
9. Sudoriferous glands are:
   a. coiled glands
   b. endocrine glands
   c. saccular glands
   d. tubular glands.
10. The digital cushion consists mainly of:
    a. muscle tissue
    b. epidermis
    c. dermis
    d. adipose tissue.
11. On average, how many pairs of mammary glands do cats have?
    a. two to four
    b. four to six
    c. six to eight
    d. eight to ten.
12. The tail gland plays a part in:
    a. waterproofing
    b. scent marking
    c. thermoregulation
    d. hair growth rate.

13. Hair is shed during:
    a. the anagen stage
    b. the catagen stage
    c. the telogen stage
    d. all stages.
14. Lanugo hairs are:
    a. guard hairs
    b. vibrissae
    c. topcoat hairs
    d. wool hairs.
15. The coronary border is situated:
    a. between the ungual process and the claw
    b. around mammary gland tissue
    c. between the abdominal and scrotal skin
    d. on the feline carpus.

Tip: *Why not get together with fellow students and write some more questions for each other?*

CHAPTER 13

Birds

LEARNING Objectives

This chapter will help you to revise the key features of the:

- musculoskeletal system
- feathers
- respiratory system
- digestive system.

There is a general revision section at the end of the chapter, which also incorporates some revision of the circulatory, urinary, reproductive systems and special senses.

The musculoskeletal system

To revise key points about the skeletal system see Chapter 3.

Primary differences:

- The bone cortex is thinner than in mammalian bones.
- Many long bones are hollow (pneumatic) with honeycombed struts for support.
- There are fewer joints than in mammals, with many bones fused together.
- The forelimbs have evolved into wings.
- The digital flexor tendon enables perching.
- The feet and toes are adapted for function, e.g. grasping, swimming or perching.

Activity

Exercise 13.1 Below is a diagram of an avian skeleton. From the selection, add the correct labels to the diagram.

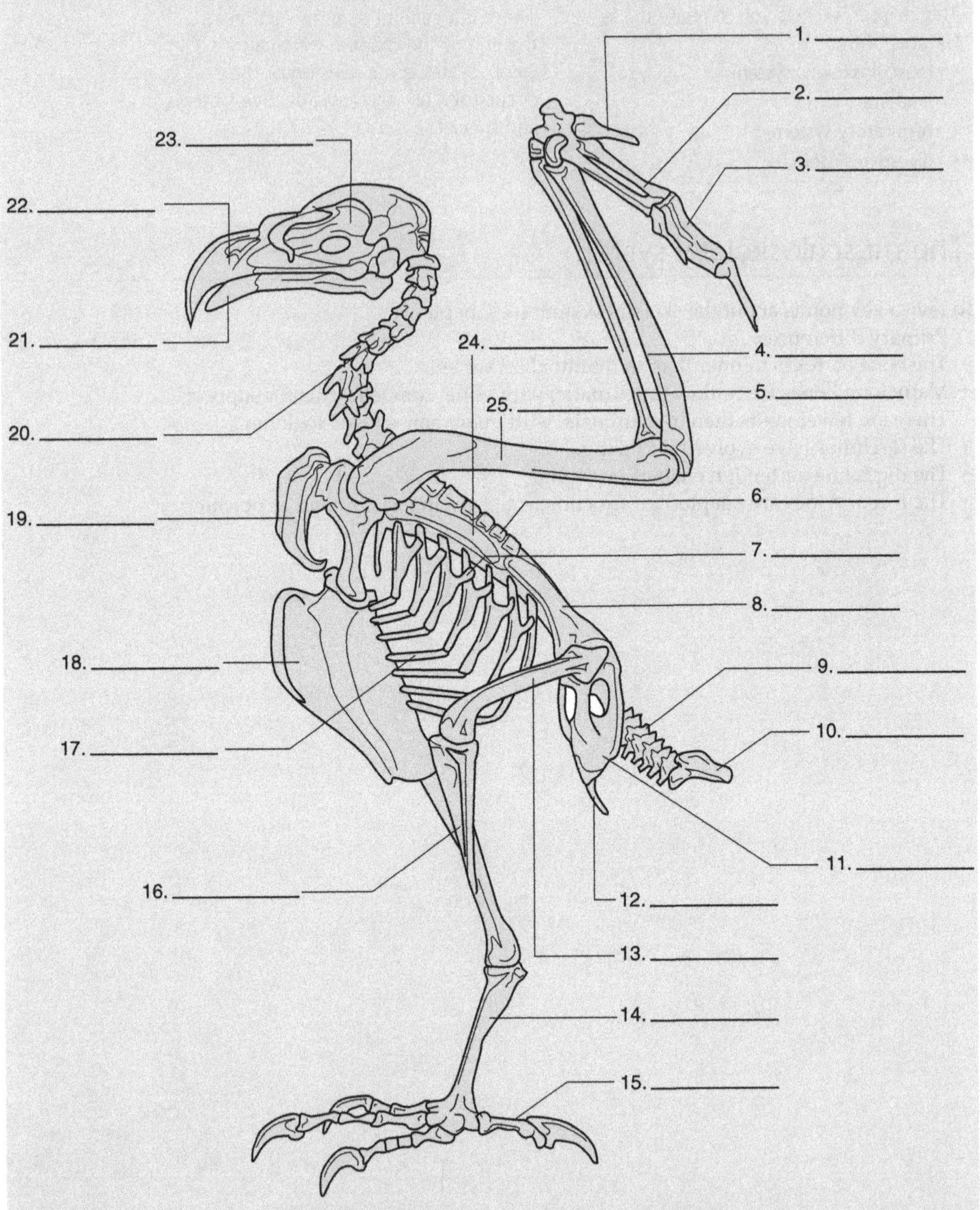

Figure 13.1 The skeleton of a typical bird.
(Adapted with permission from Aspinall & O'Reilly 2004.)

Orbit	Coccygeal vertebrae	Tarsometatarsus	Thoracic vertebrae	Pubis
Major metacarpal	Coracoid	Upper mandible	Ischium	Tibiotarsus
Uncinate process	Synsacrum	Femur	Complete rib	Ulna
Pygostyle	Cervical vertebrae	Alula (first digit)	Sternum	Second digit
Humerus	Hallux	Radius	Lower mandible	Scapula

Feathers

Key Points:

1. Feathers develop from epidermal cells
2. They are made of the protein keratin
3. Secretions from the preen gland keep the feathers waterproof
4. The feathers must be intact and clean in order to function, e.g. flight, insulation.
5. There are four types of feather:
   a. primary and contour
   b. semiplume
   c. down
   d. filoplume.

Activity

On a large piece of paper, draw the different types of feather, paying particular attention to the shape of the barbs and barbules.

Respiratory system

Key Points:

1. Birds have no diaphragm dividing the abdominal and thoracic areas, therefore they only have one body cavity.
2. The lungs are fairly rigid and do not expand as they fill with air.
3. All free spaces in the body cavity and the major bones contain air sacs enabling the bird to exchange gases on inhalation and inspiration. This makes the respiratory system extremely efficient.

Study

It is important to know where the airsacs are located in order to facilitate safe handling and administration of medication. List the name and location of the major airsacs in the body and bones.

Digestive system

Key Points:

1. Birds have a beak instead of teeth. The shape varies according to the diet, e.g. a parrot's hooked bill is adapted for cracking open nuts, fruits and seeds.
2. The crop is an extension of the oesophagus. It primarily acts as a storage organ.
3. The stomach is divided into two parts:
   a. glandular proventriculus for chemical digestion
   b. muscular ventriculus (gizzard) for mechanical digestion.
4. The gall bladder is not present in all species.
5. The paired caecae vary according to diet, e.g. ducks have large caecae for fermenting vegetation whereas the caecae of hawks are rudimentary.
6. The cloaca is the terminal opening of the digestive, urinary and reproductive tracts.

Activity

Exercise 13.2 Below is a diagram of the avian digestive tract. From the selection, add the correct labels to the diagram.

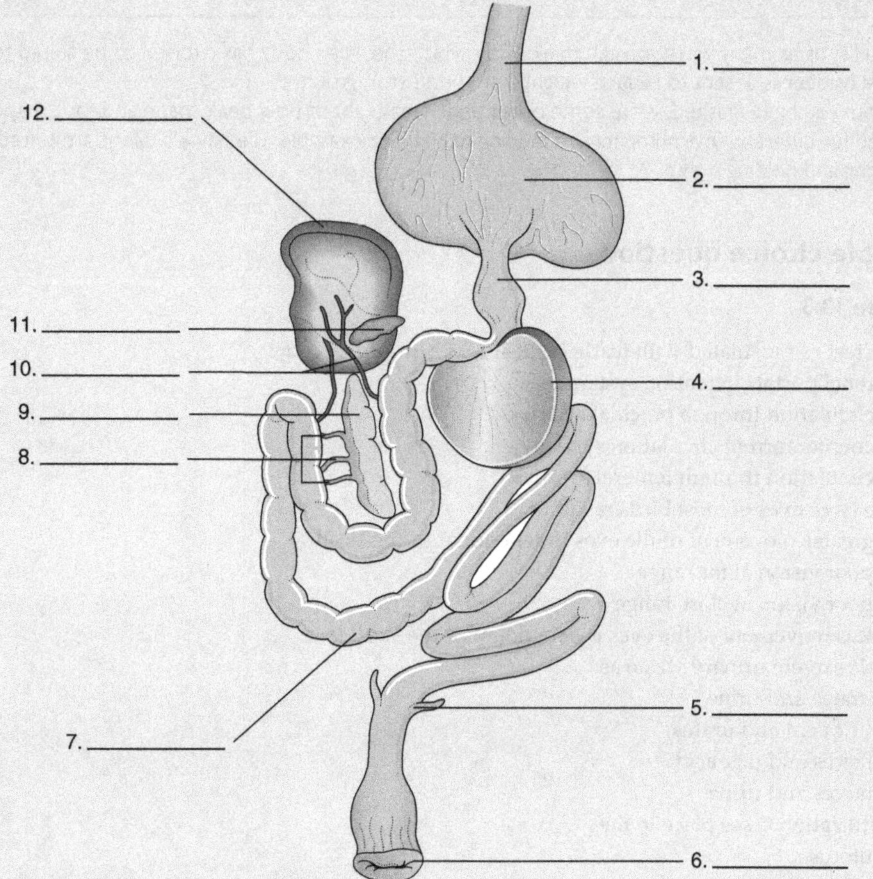

Figure 13.2 The digestive system of the pigeon.
(Adapted with permission from Aspinall & O'Reilly 2004.)

Crop	Caecum/caecae	Spleen	Ventriculus (gizzard)	Proventriculus	Oesophagus
Bile ducts	Intestine	Pancreas	Liver	Cloaca	Pancreatic ducts

General revision

Activity

Make a list of as many ways you can think of by which the avian body has evolved to be suited to flight, e.g. the bladder is absent to reduce weight from urine storage.

When you have finished, write some notes underneath about how beak shape and foot shape are adapted for different environments and feeding habits. For example, the hawk's talons are suited for capturing and holding prey.

Multiple choice questions

Exercise 13.3

1. For feet not insulated with feathers, heat loss is minimized by:
   a. renal portal circulation system
   b. circulation through brachial arteries
   c. countercurrent circulation system
   d. circulation through femoral arteries.
2. The large eyes of most birds result in:
   a. greater movement of the eyes independent of the skull
   b. poor vision at far range
   c. poor vision at close range
   d. less movement of the eyes independent of the skull.
3. Birds excrete urinary waste as:
   a. urates and urine
   b. uric acid and urates
   c. faeces and uric acid
   d. faeces and urine.
4. Fertilization takes place in the:
   a. uterus
   b. isthmus
   c. magnum
   d. infundibulum.
5. In some birds:
   a. the testes enlarge during breeding season
   b. the testes are completely absent
   c. the testes are external to the body
   d. there is only one testicle that develops.

Tip: *Why not get together with fellow students and write some more questions for each other?*

CHAPTER 14

Exotic mammals

LEARNING Objectives

Much exotic mammal anatomy and physiology is similar to that of the dog and cat—see the other chapters that are specific to the relevant body system to revise key points. This chapter will help you to revise the key differences of the:

- rabbit
- small rodent
- cavy
- chinchilla
- rat and mouse.

There is a general revision section at the end of the chapter, which also incorporates some revision of ferrets.

The rabbit

Key Points:

1. Rabbits are lagomorphs. They differ from rodents in that they have two pairs of upper incisors.
2. Rabbits are herbivorous prey animals.
3. Bone density of a rabbit is less than that of a dog or cat, making them more prone to fracture.
4. The radius and ulna and also the tibia and fibula are completely fused.
5. The teeth are open rooted so they grow continually.
6. There are no canine teeth.
7. The jaw action is circular so the premolars and molars can grind food against their horizontal surfaces.
8. Rabbits are unable to vomit due to the position of the cardiac sphincter.
9. The caecum is large and well developed to enable digest large quantities of vegetation.
10. Rabbits produce two types of faeces:
    a. hard fibrous pellets
    b. soft pellets or caecotrophs.
11. Urine colour and clarity vary according to diet.
12. In the buck, the inguinal canal so that the testes can be retracted into the abdominal cavity.
13. The male has no nipples.
14. The female is an induced ovulator and has a bicornate uterus with no body. Each uterine horn has a separate cervix.

Activity

Prepare a five-minute presentation entitled: 'What happens to a blade of grass when a rabbit eats it?' Your audience could be friends, family or fellow students. When you have finished, invite questions from the floor!

Small rodents

Key Points:

1. There are three main groups of small rodents:
   a. myomorphs—includes rats, mice, gerbils and hamsters:
      i. open rooted incisors
      ii. monogastric omnivores
      iii. unable to vomit
      iv. no large caecum (unlike herbivores)
      v. polyoestrus spontaneous ovulators
      vi. testes are external (with the exception of the Chinese hamster)
      vii. hamsters have a large stomach for cellulose breakdown
      viii. there is no gallbladder in the rat
      ix. they produce altricial young.
   b. hystricomorphs—cavies (guinea pigs) and chinchillas:
      i. monogastric herbivores
      ii. they have a large caecum (cavies more so than chinchillas)
      iii. they are coprophagic
      iv. polyoestrus spontaneous ovulators
      v. they produce precocial young
      vi. guinea pigs need daily vitamin C
      vii. the male chinchilla has no scrotum
      viii. the female chinchilla has a bicornate uterus with no body. Each uterine horn has a separate cervix.
   c. sciuromorph—chipmunks:
      i. monogastric omnivores
      ii. chipmunks have similar dentition and digestive tract to the myomorph
      iii. polyoestrus spontaneous ovulators.

General revision

Activity

Design a chart describing the differences between the three types of small rodent. Include such things as:

- age of sexual maturity
- gestation period
- litter size
- altricial or precocial young
- diet
- dental formula.

Multiple choice questions

Exercise 14.1

1. The rodent that is 'solitary' is the:
   a. chinchilla
   b. hamster
   c. gerbil
   d. cavy.
2. The small mammal that is an induced ovulator is the:
   a. gerbil
   b. rabbit
   c. cavy
   d. rat.
3. The small mammal that produces precocial young is the:
   a. rat
   b. rabbit
   c. hamster
   d. chinchilla.
4. The small mammal with a gestation period similar to the dog and cat is the:
   a. cavy
   b. rabbit
   c. mouse
   d. chinchilla.
5. The dental formula for a ferret is:
   a. [I1/1, C0/0, PM0/0, M3/3] x 2 =16 total
   b. [I1/1, C0/0, PM1/1, M3/3] x 2 =20 total
   c. [I2/1, C0/0, PM3/2, M3/3] x 2 =28 total
   d. [I3/3, C1/1, PM 3/3, M1/2] x 2 = 34 total.

Tip: *Why not get together with fellow students and write some more questions for each other?*

CHAPTER 15 Reptiles

LEARNING Objectives

Much anatomy and physiology is similar among reptilian species. This chapter will help you to revise some similarities and differences of reptiles including:

- general anatomy of most reptiles
- anatomical and physiological differences of:
  - tortoises, terrapins and turtles
  - lizards
  - snakes.

There is a general revision section at the end of the chapter.

General anatomy of most reptiles

Key Points:

1. Reptiles:
   a. are ectothermic
   b. have a three chambered heart
   c. have a renal portal system
   d. have no diaphragm dividing the abdominal and thoracic areas, therefore they only have one body cavity
   e. are oviparous or ovoviviparous
   f. are covered by scales or plates
   g. are classified into four orders:
      i. hynchocephalia—the rare tuatara
      ii. crocodilia—crocodiles and alligators
      iii. chelonia—tortoises, terrapins and turtles
      iv. squamata—lizards and snakes.

Primary anatomical and physiological differences

Key Points:

1. Tortoises, terrapins and turtles:
   a. skeleton similar to other vertebrates but with a rigid outer shell
   b. pelvic and pectoral girdles are encased within the rib cage
   c. the upper vertebrae form parts of the shell
   d. the shell is divided into the:
      i. carapace—upper portion
      ii. plastron—lower portion
   e. respiration is aided by movement of the head and limbs rather than the body wall
   f. they have a horny beak instead of teeth.

2. Lizards:
   a. skeleton similar to other vertebrates but with no sternum
   b. the teeth are regularly shed and replaced
   c. some species have a transparent lower eyelid
   d. they have a large ventral tail vein
   e. in some species, the tail can be shed as a defence mechanism (autotomy)
   f. females have two ovaries and oviducts but no uterus.
3. Snakes:
   a. skeleton similar to other vertebrates but with many vertebrae and ribs but no sternum or limbs
   b. the left lung is small or absent
   c. they have a kinetic skull enabling them to swallow large prey
   d. the teeth are constantly replaced, some species have fangs and venom
   e. the upper and lower eyelids are fused to form a spectacle over the eye
      the tongue is used to smell/taste the environment
   f. some species have heat sensitive pits on the upper jaw to detect prey
   g. snakes have no bladder
   h. males have a penis with two tips (hemipenes)
   i. some female snakes only have one ovary and oviduct.

General revision

Activity

Design a chart describing the differences between the chelonian, lizards and snakes. Include such things as:

- presence of diaphragm
- number of functional lungs
- presence of bladder
- dentition.

Why not also add birds, mammals and fish to your chart to assist in your understanding?

Multiple choice questions

Exercise 15.1

1. The three chambered reptilian heart has:
   a. one atrium and two ventricles
   b. three atria
   c. two atria and one ventricle
   d. three ventricles.
2. The renal portal system transports blood directly from the:
   a. gastrointestinal tract to the kidney
   b. kidney to the hindlimbs and tail
   c. hindlimbs and tail to the kidney
   d. kidney to the gastrointestinal tract.

3. Ecdysis is:
   a. severe oral infection
   b. shedding of the integument
   c. the condition of being 'egg-bound'
   d. the reptilian thermoregulatory mechanism.
4. Sexual dimorphism is the:
   a. ability of some reptiles to reproduce without mating
   b. determination of gender according to nest temperature
   c. differing appearance of the male and female of the same species
   d. same external appearance of the male and female of the same species.
5. Each individual plate on the shell of a chelonian is called a:
   a. carapace
   b. plastron
   c. scute
   d. beak.
6. Jacobsen's organ is found in the:
   a. roof of the mouth
   b. tip of the tongue
   c. tip of the tail
   d. canal of the ear.

Tip: *Why not get together with fellow students and write some more questions for each other?*

CHAPTER 16

The horse

LEARNING Objectives

Much equine anatomy and physiology is similar to that of the dog and this chapter is designed to assist revision of the differences between these two species. This chapter will help you to revise the key differences between canine and equine anatomy of the:

- skeletal system
- muscular system
- foot
- eye
- digestive system
- reproductive system.

There is a general revision section at the end of the chapter, which also incorporates some revision of the blood vascular, respiratory and urinary systems.

The skeletal system

To revise key points about the skeletal system see Chapter 3.

Primary differences:

- The vertebral column consists of approximately 54 individual vertebrae.
- The horse has 18 ribs. The first eight ribs are the sternal ribs and the final 10 ribs are the asternal ribs.
- The radius and ulna are fused and weight is borne on the central digit (the third metacarpal/tarsal) and then carried up the strong single fused bone.
- The central digit is encased in a hoof while the outer toes are reduced to vestigial appendages that no longer reach the ground.

Activity

Exercise 16.1 Below is a diagram of an equine skeleton. From the selection, add the correct labels to the diagram.

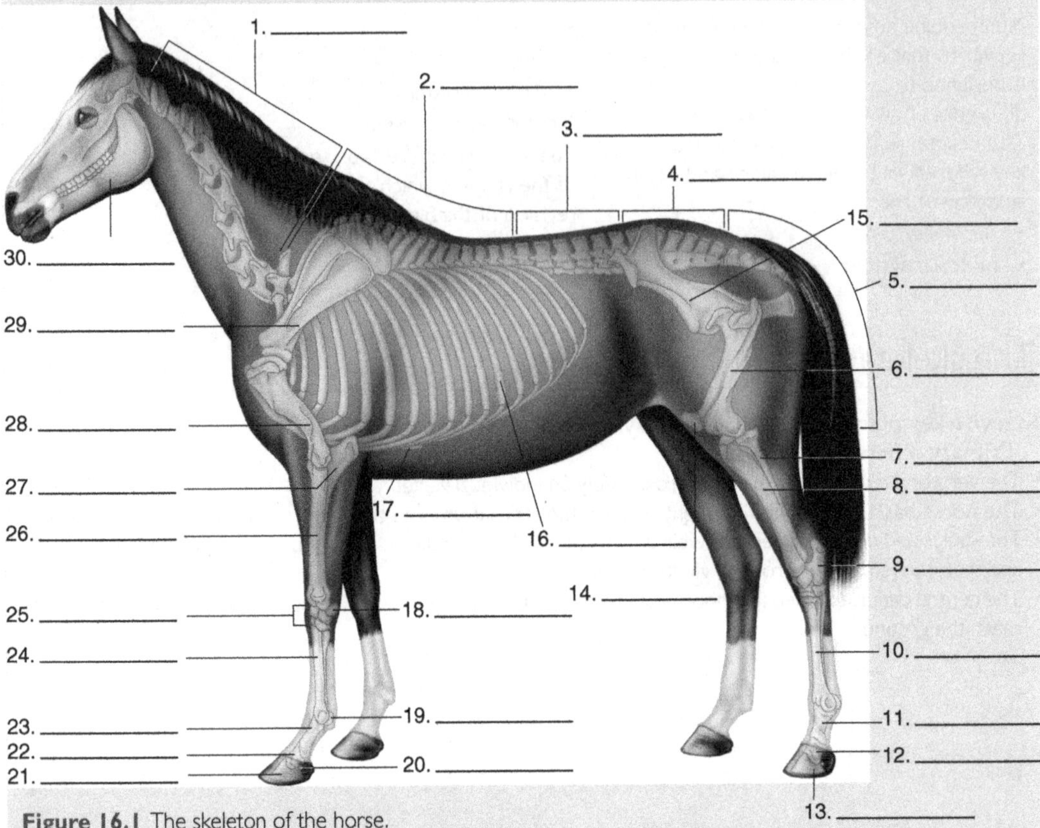

Figure 16.1 The skeleton of the horse.
(Adapted with permission from Aspinall 2006.)

Cervical vertebrae	Proximal sesamoid	Radius	Patella	Proximal phalanx hindlimb
Humerus	Thoracic vertebrae	Carpus	Sacrum	Middle phalanx forelimb
Metatarsal bones	Proximal phalanx forelimb	Middle phalanx hindlimb	Metacarpus	Tarsal bones
Distal phalanx	Scapula	Fibula	Pelvis	Coccygeal vertebrae
Distal sesamoid	Lumbar vertebrae	Ulna	Distal phalanx hindlimb	Skull
Rib	Accessory carpal bone	Tibia	Femur	Sternum

Look it up

Exercise 16.2 Complete the chart below by writing the correct numbers of each type of vertebra in the boxes.

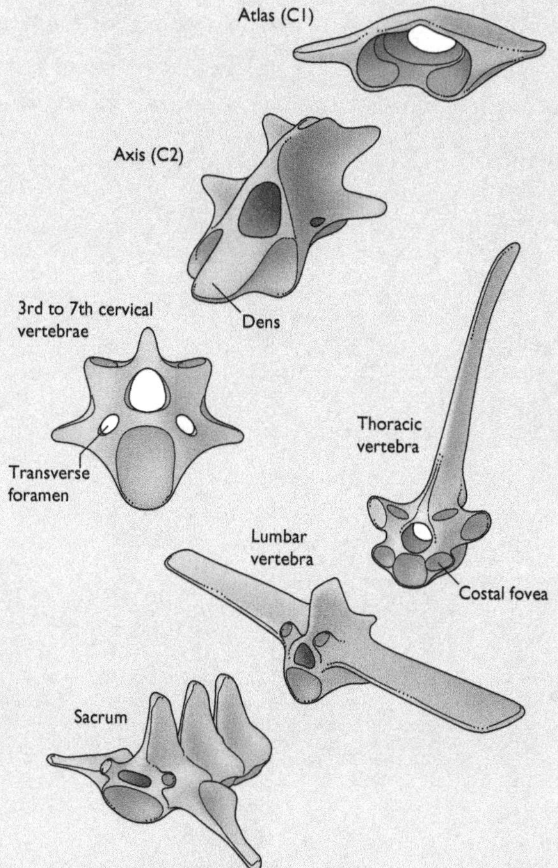

Figure 16.2 The shape of each equine vertebral type.
(Adapted with permission from Aspinall & Cappello 2009.)

Cervical	Thoracic	Lumbar	Sacral	Coggyceal
(1)	(2)	(3) (fused)	(4)	(5)

What am I?

Exercise 16.3 Write the common names for the structures listed below in the box provided

Carpus	(1)
Third metacarpal/tarsal	(2)
Metacarpals II and IV	(3)
First phalanx	(4)
Second phalanx	(5)
Third phalanx	(6)
Metacarpophalangeal joint	(7)
Distal sesamoid	(8)
Distal interphalangeal joint	(9)
Proximomedial interphalangeal joint	(10)

The muscular system

To revise key points about muscles see Chapter 4.

Activity

Below is a diagram of the superficial muscles of the horse. To make a jigsaw puzzle follow the steps below.

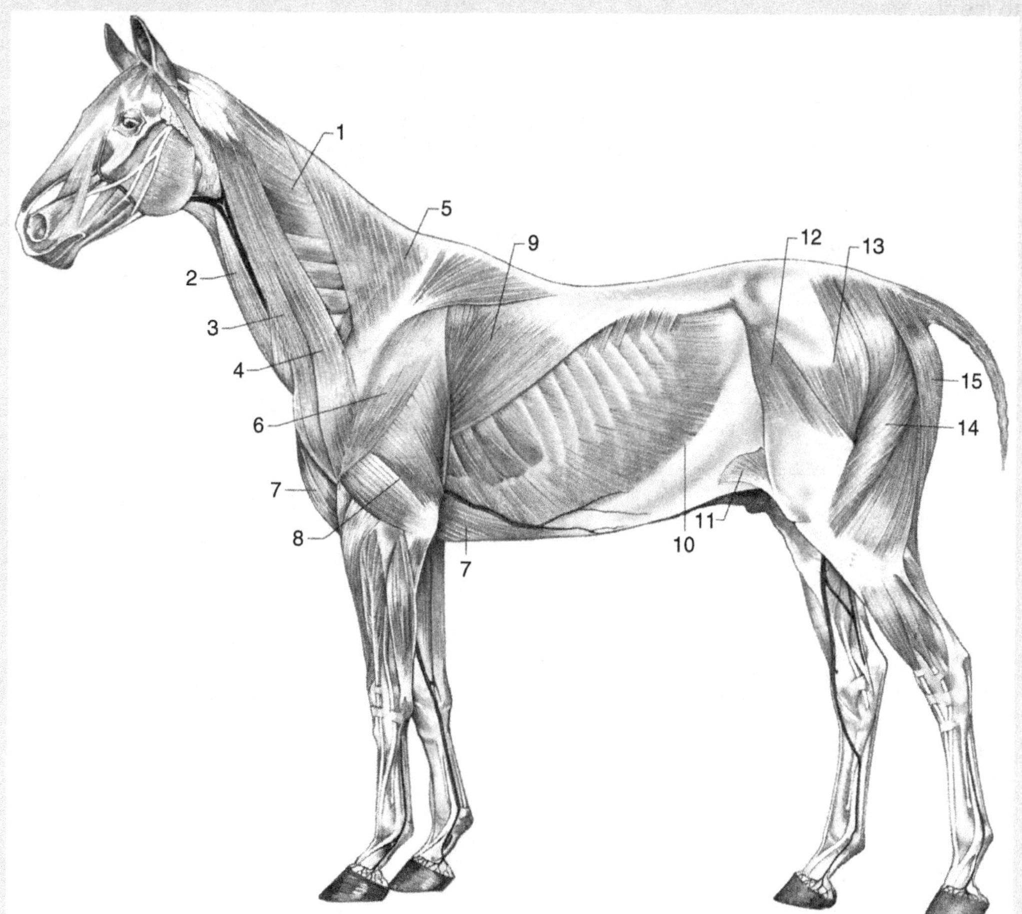

Figure 16.3 The superficial muscles of the horse.
(Adapted with permission from Dyce, Sack & Wensing 2002.),

1. Photocopy the diagram, enlarging it if necessary
2. Colour in and label the photocopy
3. Cut out each individual muscle
4. Keep the pieces safe! You can use the pieces several times to help you learn muscular anatomy.

Structure of the foot and hoof

To revise key points about the skeletal and muscular systems see Chapters 3 and 4, respectively.

Activity

Exercise 16.4 Below are diagrams of the equine foot. From the selection, add the correct labels to the diagrams.

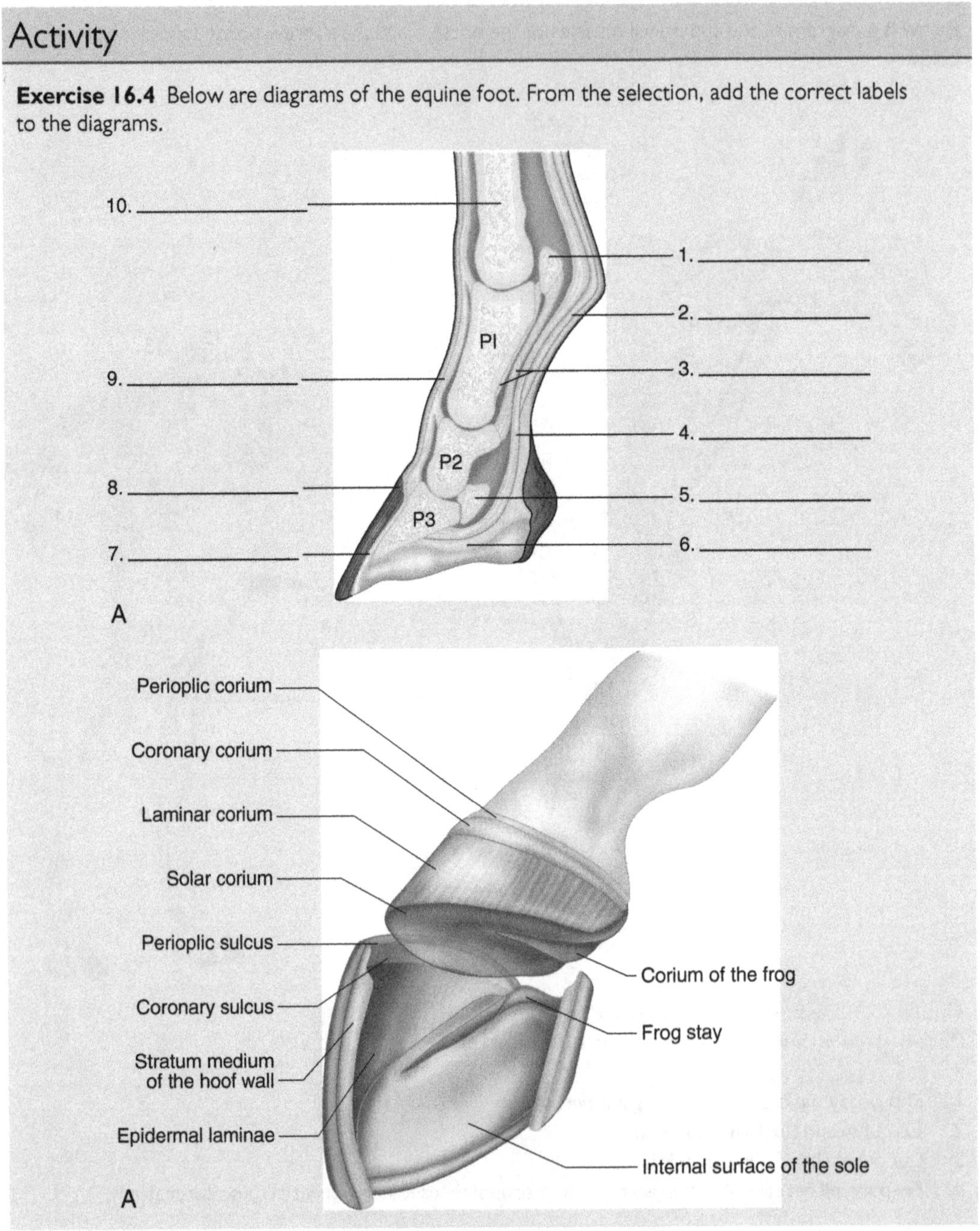

(Continued)

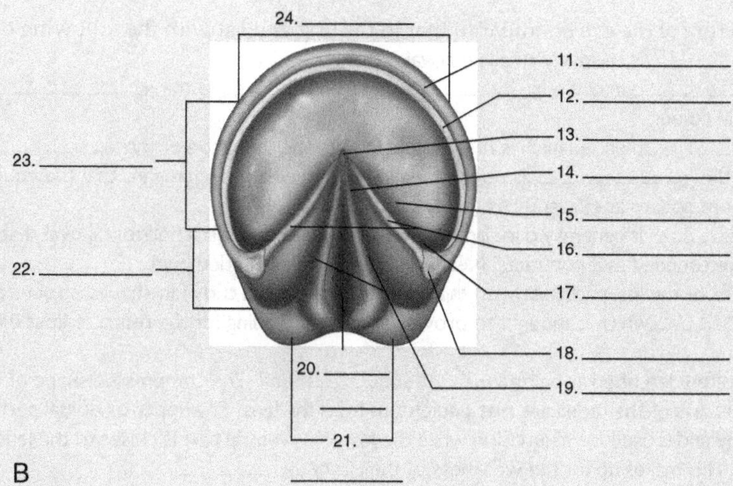

Figure 16.4 Parts of the equine foot. A. Lateral view of the distal part of the forelimb. B. Weight-bearing surface.
(Adapted with permission from Aspinall 2006.)

Metacarpal III	Toe	Bulbs	Water line	Digital cushion
White line	Point of frog	Bars	Proximal sesamoid bone	Seat of corn (angle of heel)
Superficial digital flexor tendon	Cleft or frog	Hoof wall	Buttress of heel	Quarters
White line	Commissures	Frog	Extensor tendon	Sole
Deep digital flexor tendon	Sesamoidian ligaments	Distal sesamoid (navicular bone)	Heel	

The eye

To revise key points about the eye see Chapter 5.

Fill in the gaps

Exercise 16.5 Complete the paragraph by filling in the gaps using the correct words from the selection below.

- retina
- optic disc
- Tapetum lucidum
- muscle
- ramp
- ciliary
- iris
- corpora nigra
- cornea
- light
- lens
- choroid

The basic structure of the eye is similar to that in the dog and cat with the following differences:

- The (1)____________is relatively small and oval.
- The (2)____________contains a (3)____________which lies dorsal to the (4)____________and is bluish–green in colour.
- The (5)____________muscle which is responsible for altering the shape of the (6)____________to focus images on to the (7)____________is poorly developed and weak which means that the equine lens is unable to accommodate as efficiently as the dog and the cat.
- The (8)____________is generally dark brown and the pupil within it is a horizontal oval shape but becomes more rounded as it contracts. Newborn foals have a rounded pupil.
- On the margins of the iris, particularly on the upper part there is a curly fan-shaped structure called the (9)____________which is thought to provide additional shading for the retina to limit the entry of (10)____________.
- The retina is often described as being a (11)____________retina. The compressed shape of the eyeball means that all parts of the retina are **not** equidistant from the lens. The upper or dorsal part of the retina is further away and is used for near vision while the lower or ventral part is closer to the lens and is used for far vision. This makes up for the weakness of the ciliary (12)____________.

The digestive system

To revise key points about digestion see Chapter 9.

Primary differences:

- The horse is an herbivorous prey species.
- Anatomy and physiology of the digestive tract are similar to those of the dog and cat but the tract is proportionally much longer as fibre takes longer to break down.
- Horses have two sets of teeth during their lifetime. The tooth types are:
  - incisors—responsible for cutting grass as it is taken into the mouth. There are twelve incisors—six in each jaw—which are categorized according to their position as centrals, laterals and corners. See Figure 16.5.
  - canines—these are rudimentary teeth and often fail to erupt in mares, although they may develop in 25% of mares. In stallions these *'tushes'* develop at around the age of five years, and they cause no problem. They erupt in the space, known as the diastema, between the incisors and cheek teeth.
  - premolars and molars (cheek teeth)—flattened teeth primarily used for chewing and grinding up the food. In each jaw there are six premolars and six molars. In addition *wolf teeth* (see Figure 16.5) may develop at eighteen months to five years of age. These are small vestigial teeth that develop in front of the premolars usually in the upper jaw.
  - equine teeth are described as being *hypsodontal,* i.e. they do not have a layer of enamel over the top or occlusal surface. During life the enamel and the softer dentine provide an efficient grinding surface which wears down as the teeth grow and the animal ages. These changes are described variously as marks, stars and grooves and they can be used to give a rough indication as to the age of the individual horse
- All the teeth grow continuously while the occlusal surfaces are worn down by as much as 2–3 mm a year by the mastication process.
- The cardiac sphincter does not allow matter to return from the stomach back to the oesphagus, so ingested toxins must pass through the whole system.
- Unlike the dog and cat, the horse has no gall bladder.

- The horse is classed as a hindgut fermenter, i.e. the caecum and colon are adapted to provide a chamber in which microbial digestion of cellulose (complex carbohydrates) takes place.
- The micro-organisms consisting mainly of bacteria and protozoa are specific to the horse's diet and they are highly sensitive to dietary change.

Activity

Exercise 16.6 Below are diagrams of the dentition of a horse. Label the different types and numbers of teeth and the diastema.

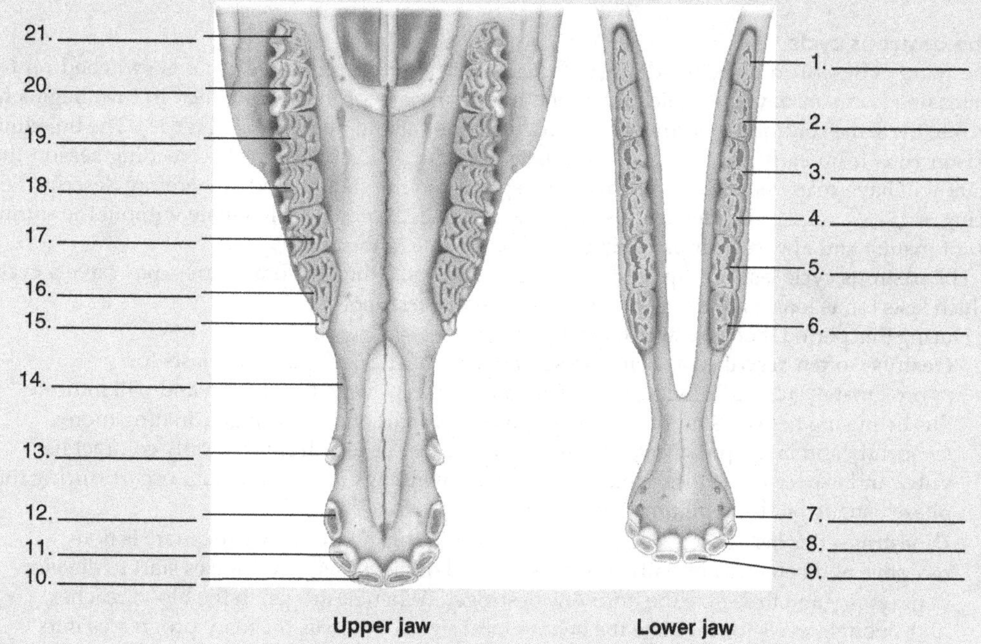

Figure 16.5 Teeth in the upper and lower jaw of a 4.5-year-old horse.
(Adapted with permission from Aspinall 2006.)

The reproductive system

To revise key points about reproduction see Chapter 11.

Primary differences:

- The testes of the colt foal may be present in the scrotum at birth or may descend within the first two weeks of life.
- The accessory glands are responsible for the production of seminal fluid. There are three sets of glands: prostate gland, seminal vesicles or vesicular gland and bulbo-urethral glands.
- There is no os penis in the male horse.
- In the mare, the ovaries are largely inactive until the mare reaches sexual maturity at around one to two years of age.
- The mare is uniparous, i.e. naturally gives birth to one foal at a time.
- The two mammary glands or udders of the mare are small and lie on the ventral surface of the caudal abdomen and cranial part of the pelvis.

Fill in the gaps

Exercise 16.7 Complete the paragraphs by filling in the gaps using the correct words from the selection below.

- 3–5
- 14–16
- Seasonally polyoestrous
- Long-day breeder
- Ovulation
- On heat
- Spring
- Spontaneous ovulator
- Oestrus
- Anoestrous
- 17–21
- Summer

The oestrous cycle

The mare is described as being a (1)____________, i.e. her reproductive cycle is switched on by increasing hours of daylight which affect the hypothalamus of the brain which in turn begins to secrete the same controlling hormones that occur in the cat and dog (see Chapter 11). The breeding season runs from early (2)____________to late (3)____________. Within the breeding season the mare will have many periods of oestrus or receptivity to the stallion and is therefore described as being (4)____________. The mare is also a (5)____________, i.e. she will ovulate without the stimulus of mating and always at approximately the same time of the cycle.

The oestrous cycle lasts for up to (6)____________days, although some mares may have a cycle which lasts for as long as 35 days—there is individual variation.

During this period there are two distinct phases:

1. **Oestrus**—often described as being 'in season' or '(7)____________'. This lasts for approximately (8)____________days. The mare is receptive to the stallion and will indicate this by raising her tail, standing with her hind legs apart and squatting, urinating more frequently and in the presence of a stallion or a 'teaser', she will rhythmically contract her vulva and expose her clitoris which is known as 'winking'. (9)____________occurs during this phase usually on the penultimate or last day.
2. **Dioestrus**—this lasts for (10)____________days and during this phase the mare is non-receptive and behaves normally. Towards the end of dioestrus new follicles start to develop in the ovary and to secrete the hormone oestrogen. When oestrogen in the blood reaches high enough levels to stimulate the behavioural signs of oestrus the mare progresses into (11)____________again.

During the shorter daylight hours of the winter months the oestrous cycles cease and the mare is described as being (12)____________.

General revision

Activity

Make a list of as many ways you can think of by which the equine body has evolved to be suited to its natural environment and lifestyle. When you have finished, write some notes underneath about how modern ideas about care and use of horses can cause problems. For example, how can being stable-kept affect a horse's digestive function?

Multiple choice questions

Exercise 16.8

1. The tendon whose function is to extend the pastern joint and the toe is the:
   a. Deep digital flexor tendon
   b. Superficial digital flexor tendon
   c. Common digital extensor tendon
   d. Lateral digital extensor tendon.
2. The structure that prevents overextension of the fetlock is the:
   a. suspensory ligament
   b. check ligament
   c. suspensory apparatus
   d. stay apparatus.
3. Pulse rate is measured at the:
   a. facial artery
   b. jugular vein
   c. femoral artery
   d. lingual vein.
4. Normal heart rate of a resting horse is:
   a. 25–42 beats per minute
   b. 42–120 beats per minute
   c. 120–220 beats per minute
   d. 220–240 beats per minute.
5. The equine kidney differs from that of a dog in that:
   a. there is only one kidney in the horse
   b. the left and right kidneys are different shapes
   c. the right kidney is more cranial than the left
   d. the kidneys produce urates rather than urine.
6. Horses produce urine at a rate of approximately:
   a. 2 ml/kg/day
   b. 20 ml/kg/day
   c. 200 ml/kg/day
   d. 2000 ml/kg/day.

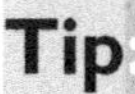

Why not get together with fellow students and write some more questions for each other?

Answers to exercises

1 Body composition and cells

1.1. **1** Organic pertains to chemical compounds containing carbon. **2** Inorganic pertains to chemical compounds that do not contain carbon.

1.2. **1** 60–70; **2** higher; **3** lower; **4** obese; **5** compartments; **6** intracellular; **7** extracellular; **8** interstitial; **9** intravascular; **10** respiratory; **11** cutaneous; **12** gastrointestinal; **13** lacrimation; **14** urinary; **15** insensible.

1.3. **1** 20; **2** 20; **3** 10–20; **4** 20; **5** 50–60.

1.4. **1–10**; **3–8**; **5–2**; **7–4**; **9–6**.

1.5. **1** Na; **2**+; **3** Cl; **4**–; **5** K; **6**+; **7** Ca; **8**+; **9** P; **10**–; **11** Mg; **12**+.

1.6. **1** 38.3–38.7°C; **2** 38.0–38.5°C; **3** 7.4; **4** 7.4; **5** 1–2 ml/kg/24 hrs; **6** 1–2 ml/kg/24 hrs; **7** 1.015—1.045; **8** 1.020—1.060; **9** 20 ml/kg/24 hrs; **10** 20 ml/kg/24 hrs; **11**, approx 180/100 **12**, approx 180/100.

1.7. **1–6**; **3–18**; **5–2**; **7–12**; **9–8**; **11–14**; **13–16**; **15–4**; **17–10**.

1.8. **1** membranes; **2** concentrated; **3** equalize; **4** diffusion; **5** water; **6** less; **7** more; **8** higher; **9** gradient; **10** isotonic; **11** hypertonic; **12** hypotonic.

1.9. **1–4**; **3–8**; **5–2**; **7–10**; **9–6**.

1.10. 3; 8; 1; 11; 6; 10; 5; 9; 4; 2; 7.

1.11. **1** everywhere but the gonads; **2** gonads; **3** one round; **4** two rounds; **5** two; **6** four; **7** diploid; **8** haploid; **9** does not occur; **10** occurs; **11** identical; **12** non-identical.

1.12. **1** b; **2** c; **3** b; **4** c; **5** c; **6** d; **7** b; **8** a.

1.13. **1** ABDOMINAL; **2** INORGANIC; **3** ACIDOSIS; **4** HYDROGEN; **5** CELLS; **6** FORTY; **7** MINERALS; **8** PH; **9** OSMOSIS; **10** SODIUM; **11** URINE; **12** EXTRACELLULAR; **13** CALCIUM; **14** BLOOD; **15** ION.

1.14. **1** a; **2** b; **3** c; **4** c; **5** a; **6** d; **7** a; **8** c; **9** a; **10** a; **11** b; **12** d; **13** d; **14** c; **15** a.

1.15. **1** ENDOCYTOSIS; **2** REDUCTION; **3** LYSOSOMES; **4** TELOPHASE; **5** SODIUM; **6** ATP; **7** POLAR; **8** ACTIVE; **9** FOUR; **10** NUCLEUS; **11** GONADS.

2 Body tissues and cavities

2.1. **1** basement; **2** alveoli; **3** liver; **4** cilia; **5** goblet; **6** oviduct; **7** genital; **8** keratin; **9** foot pads; **10** ureters; **11** urine; **12** reduced.

2.2. **1** no general name; **2** hormones; **3** via a duct; **4** via the bloodstream; **5** near site of action; **6** not necessarily near site of action.

2.3. Hyaline 3, 4, 7; Fibro 5, 6; Elastic 1, 2, 8.

2.4. Mediastinum, heart, trachea, oesophagus, thymus, bronchi, lung tissue, lymph nodes and vessels, blood vessels, nerves.

2.5. Liver, gall bladder, spleen, oesophagus, stomach, small intestine, large intestine, pancreas, (in the female: ovaries, oviducts, uterus), (in the male: spermatic cord, prostate), ureters, urinary bladder, urethra, lymph nodes and vessels, blood vessels, nerves. (NB Kidneys are retroperitoneal.)

2.6. **1** a; **2** d; **3** b; **4** b; **5** c.

2.7. Across **1** ENDOTHELIUM; **5** BONE; **9** NERVE; **11** CUBOIDAL; **12** KERATIN; **13** SCARS. Down **1** EMBRYONIC; **2** DENSE; **3** HORMONE; **4** MYO; **6** URETER; **7** TENDON; **8** AREOLAR; **10** HYALINE.

2.8. **1** b; **2** b; **3** d; **4** b; **5** b; **6** d; **7** b; **8** d.

3 The skeletal system

3.1. **1** Haversian canal; **2** Osteocyte; **3** Lacuna; **4** Lamellae; **5** Calcified matrix.

3.2. (a) Cartilage model in fetus; (b) Ossification begins from primary centre of ossification in shaft (diaphysis); (c) Ossification in shaft continues. Secondary centres of ossification appear in epiphyses; (d) Ossification continues in diaphysis and epiphyses. Osteoclasts begin to break down bone in shaft to form marrow cavity; (e) First growth plate fuses. Medullary cavity continues into epiphysis. Growth is only now possible at proximal growth plate; (f) Proximal growth plate fuses. Bone growth ceases.

3.3. **1** Epiphysis; **2** Diaphysis; **3** Hyaline articular cartilage; **4** Compact bone; **5** Epiphyseal lines; **6** Cancellous bone trabeculae; **7** Metaphysis; **8** Diaphysis (shaft); **9** Compact bone; **10** Marrow cavity (medullary cavity); **11** Fibrous layer; **12** Periosteum osteogenic layer.

3.4. **1–18**; **3–10**; **5–16**; **7–12**; **9–8**; **11–2**; **13–6**; **15–4**; **17–20**; **19–14**.

3.5. **1** C1, atlas; **2** C2, axis; **3** Ligamentum nuchae; **4** T1 first thoracic vertebra; **5** L1 first lumbar vertebra; **6** Sacrum; **7** Cy1 first vertebra (coccygeal); **8** Os coxae (pelvis); **9** Calcaneus (point of hock); **10** Metatarsal bones; **11** Tarsal bones; **12** Fibula; **13** Tibia; **14** Patella; **15** Femur; **16** Caudal end (xiphoid) of sternum; **17** Metacarpal bones; **18** Proximal, middle, and distal phalanges; **19** Carpal bones; **20** Ulna; **21** Radius; **22** Olecranon (point of elbow); **23** Humerus; **24** Cranial end of sternum (manubrium); **25** Scapula; **26** C7 last cervical vertebra.

3.6. **1** 7; **2** 13; **3** 7; **4** 3 (fused); **5** 15–21 (average).

3.7. **1–8**; **3–10**; **5–12**; **7–2**; **9–4**; **11–6**.

3.8. **1** Wing of ilium; **2** Ilium; **3** Pubis; **4** Obturator foramen; **5** Ischium; **6** Pubic symphysis; **7** Ischial tuberosity; **8** Acetabulum; **9** Ischium; **10** Obturator foramen; **11** Pubis; **12** Wing of ilium.

3.9. **1** radius; **2** femur; **3** tibia; **4** humerus; **5** fibula; **6** ulna.

3.10. **1** Radius; **2** 2 rows of carpal bones; **3** Proximal phalanx of digit 1 (sometimes labelled metacarpal 1); **4** Medial phalanx of digit 2; **5** Distal phalanx of digit 3 with the ungual process that forms the nail core; **6** Distal phalanges; **7** Medial phalanges; **8** Proximal phalanges; **9** 4 Metacarpal bones (numbered 2–5); **10** Ulna.

3.11. **1** Tibia; **2** Fibula; **3** Phalanges of dew claw attached to tarsus; **4** Fibular tarsalor calcaneus which makes point of hock; **5** Metatarsals; **6** Proximal phalanges; **7** Medial phalanges; **8** Distal phalanges (with ungual process).

3.12. **1** Articular cartilage; **2** Synovial membrane (inner); **3** Fibrous membrane (outer); **4** Periosteum; **5** Synovial fluid.

3.13. **1** fibrous; **2** synovial; **3** synovial; **4** cartilaginous (amphiarthrosis); **5** cartilaginous (amphiarthrosis); **6** synovial; **7** synovial; **8** cartilaginous (synarthrosis); **9** synovial.

3.14. **1** scapula, humerus; **2** humerus, radius, ulna; **3** radius, ulna, carpal bones; **4** ilium, ischium, pubis, acetabular bone, femur; **5** femur, tibia, fibula, patella, fabellae; **6** tibia, fibula, tarsal bones.

3.15. **1** d; **2** b; **3** a; **4** c; **5** b; **6** a; **7** d; **8** d; **9** a; **10** c.

3.16. **1** true; **2** false (the mandibular symphysis is a cartilaginous joint); **3** true; **4** false (there are eight sternebrae); **5** true; **6** true; **7** false (the os penis is part of the splanchnic skeleton); **8** true.

3.17. Across **6** ABDUCTION; **7** RIBCAGE; **11** OSSIFICATION; **14** ULNA; **15** DEWCLAW; **17** FEMUR; **18** STERNAL; **19** STRAW; **20** EIGHT; **21** SHOULDER; **22** LUMBAR. Down **1** INCISIVE; **2** ILIUM; **3** COSTAL; **4** ARTH; **5** HAVERSIAN; **8** BRAIN; **9** MEATUS; **10** DIAPHYSIS; **12** SCAPULA; **13** NINE; **16** CANCELLOUS.

4 The muscular system

4.1. Cardiac 7; Involuntary 1, 2, 3, 5, 8; Voluntary 4, 6, 9.

4.2. **1–4**; **3–18**; **5–10**; **7–16**; **9–14**; **11–8**; **13–2**; **15–12**; **17–6**

4.3. Aortic hiatus 1, 5, 6; Oesophageal hiatus 2, 4; Caval foramen 3.

4.4. **1–4**; **3–8**; **5–2**; **7–6**.

4.5. **1** LATISSIMUS; **2** MOTOR UNIT; **3** INTRINSIC; **4** BRACHIALIS; **5** OLECRANON; **6** INTERCOSTAL; **7** INFRASPINATUS; **8** EXTENSOR; **9** FLEXOR; **10** TENDON; **11** APONEUROSIS; **12** GLUTEAL; **13** BICEPS FEMORIS; **14** STRIATED; **15** ORIGIN; **16** QUADRICEPS; **17** CARDIAC; **18** TIBIALIS; **19** TRAPEZIUS; **20** INSERTION.

4.6. **1** b; **2** d; **3** d; **4** d; **5** c.

4.7. **1** masseter; **2** temporalis; **3** rectus abdominis; **4** biceps brachii; **5** biceps femoris.

5 The nervous system and special senses

5.1. **1** Dendrite; **2** Cell body; **3** Nucleus; **4** Axon; **5** Schwann cell; **6** Myelin sheath; **7** Axon branch (collateral axon); **8** Node of Ranvier.

5.2. **1–8**; **3–16**; **5–2**; **7–4**; **9–22**; **11–18**; **13–10**; **15–12**; **17–14**; **19–6**; **21–20**.

5.3. **1** cranial; **2** meninges; **3** four; **4** ventricles; **5** cerebrospinal fluid; **6** cerebrum; **7** two; **8** longitudinal sulcus; **9** thalamus; **10** hypothalamus; **11** temperature control; **12** pituitary gland; **13** cerebellum; **14** pons; **15** brainstem; **16** cardiovascular.

5.4. **1** Nerve to epaxial region; **2** Dorsal root ganglion; **3** Dorsal root; **4** White matter; **5** Nerve to hypaxial muscles, body wall and limbs; **6** To sympathetic chain; **7** Ventral root; **8** Central canal; **9** Grey matter.

5.5. Dura mater 3, 6, 9. Arachnoid mater 2, 5, 8. Pia mater 1, 4, 7.

5.6. **1** CSF; **2** blood plasma; **3** protein; **4** ventricles; **5** subarachnoid space; **6** central canal; **7** cushions; **8** cisterna magna; **9** atlanto-occipital.

5.7. **1–18**; **3–14**; **5–6**; **7–12**; **9–2**; **11–24**; **13–20**; **15–4**; **17–8**; **19–10**; **21–16**; **23–22**.

5.8. **1** increases; **2** decreases; **3** increases; **4** decreases; **5** constrict; **6** dilate; **7** reduces; **8** increases; **9** dilate; **10** constrict.

5.9. **1–8**; **3–14**; **5–12**; **7–6**; **9–2**; **11–10**; **13–4**.

5.10. **1** Sclera; **2** Posterior chamber; **3** Limbus; **4** Iris; **5** Pupil; **6** Cornea; **7** Anterior chamber; **8** Ciliary body; **9** Suspensory ligaments; **10** Lens; **11** Choroid; **12** Retina; **13** Optic nerve; **14** Optic disc.

5.11. **1–6**; **3–10**; **5–12**; **7–16**; **9–2**; **11–18**; **13–8**; **15–4**; **17–14**.

5.12. 4; 7; 1; 6; 8; 3; 2; 5.

5.13. **1** Auricular cartilage covered in skin; **2** Annular cartilage surrounding canal; **3** Temporal bone; **4** External acoustic meatus; **5** Auditory canal—horizontal section; **6** Specialized skin containing ceruminous glands; **7** Auditory canal—vertical section; **8** Marginal cutaneous pouch.

5.14. **1–8**; **3–12**; **5–14**; **7–2**; **9–6**; **11–10**; **13–4**; **15–16**.

5.15. **1** pinna; **2** tympanic; **3** ossicles; **4** cochlea; **5** Corti; **6** vestibulocochlear; **7** semicircular; **8** endolymph; **9** crista; **10** utricle; **11** saccule; **12** maculae.

5.16. **1** b; **2** c; **3** a; **4** a; **5** a; **6** d; **7** c; **8** b.

5.17. **Dog steps on shard of glass whilst running.** Sensory (afferent) nerve pathway is stimulated and spinal reflex is initiated, reflex causes stimulation of motor (efferent) pathway directly from spinal cord and dog withdraws foot; meanwhile sensory information reaches the brain and the dog becomes aware of injury.

Dog reaches playmates but is distracted by the smell of a nearby butcher's shop. Chemoreceptors in dog's nose detect smell and sensory (afferent) pathway sends impulses to the brain via cranial nerve, brain interprets information, motor (efferent) pathway via spinal nerves sends information to the skeletal muscles to move dog in direction of butcher's shop.

Dog reaches shop and tries to enter but butcher throws bucket of cold water over dog! Sensory nerve endings in skin detect sudden temperature change and impulses are sent to the brain via spinal nerves, brain interprets information, dog aware of unpleasant cold sensation, impulses are sent via motor (efferent) pathway to skeletal muscle to halt movement into shop.

Dog's paw starts to hurt and he limps off in the direction of home. Sensory (afferent) nerve pathway sends information to brain via spinal nerves, brain interprets information, dog becomes aware of pain, information is sent via motor (efferent) pathway to alter gait and move in direction of home.

5.18. **1** c; **2** a; **3** c; **4** d; **5** c.

5.19. **1** b; **2** d; **3** c; **4** a; **5** b; **6** b; **7** d; **8** d; **9** c; **10** b.

5.20. Across **1** AQUEOUS; **3** TEAR; **5** DILATE; **8** TAPETUM; **10** OPTIC; **11** PUPIL; **13** LACRIMAL; **14** IRIS; **16** FOCAL; **17** SUSPENSORY. Down **1** ANTERIOR; **2** SCLERA; **4** RODS; **5** DOG; **6** RETINA; **7** MEDIAL; **9** MEIBOMIAN; **12** ORBIT; **13** LIMBUS; **15** FOUR.

5.21. **1** a; **2** b; **3** c; **4** d; **5** d; **6** c.

5.22. **1** Endolymphatic sac; **2** Utricle; **3** Saccule; **4** Auditory tube; **5** Vestibular window; **6** Tympanic bulla; **7** Stapes; **8** Incus; **9** Malleus; **10** Tympanic membrane; **11** Horizontal canal; **12** Vertical canal; **13** Pinna.

6 Endocrine system

6.1.

Area of pituitary gland	Hormone	Site of action	Function
Anterior pituitary (adenohypophysis)	FSH (follicle-stimulating hormone)	Ovarian follicles	Stimulates follicular maturation
	ACTH (adrenocorticotrophic hormone)	Adrenal cortex	Regulates adrenocortical hormone secretion
	TSH (thyroid-stimulating hormone)	Thyroid glands	Regulates uptake of iodine
	LH (luteinizing hormone)	Ovarian follicles	Stimulates development of corpus luteum
	ICSH (interstitial cell-stimulating hormone)	Seminiferous tubules	Stimulates sperm production; the male equivalent of LH
	Prolactin	Mammary glands	Stimulates milk production
	Somatotrophin	Mainly bones	Regulates growth rate
Posterior pituitary (neurohypophysis)	ADH (anti-diuretic hormone)	Renal tubules	Increases water absorption
	Oxytocin	Smooth muscles of uterus and mammary glands	Facilitates parturition

6.2. **1** increased; **2** unchanged; **3** increased; **4** unchanged; **5** poor; **6** poor; **7** poor; **8** excessive growth and tangling, poor, alopecia in areas; **9** decreases; **10** increases; **11** excitable, can be aggressive; **12** lethargic, sleep increases, gets cold easily.

6.3.

Area	Hormone produced	Target	Action
Adrenal cortex	Steroids: *mineralocorticoids (aldosterone) and gluco-corticoids (corticosterone and cortisol)*	Kidney Bloodstream; liver	Regulate electrolyte balance Increase blood glucose level
	Male/female sex hormones	Many body systems	Masculinization; feminization; sexual activity
Adrenal medulla	Adrenaline (epinephrine) Noradrenaline (norepinephrine)	CV, respiratory and nervous systems	Prepare for 'fight or flight'; increase heart rate, respiration, etc.

6.4. **1** increased; **2** lack of insulin starves cells of energy; **3** decreased; **4** lack of insulin starves cells of energy; **5** hyperglycaemia; **6** lack of insulin prevents uptake of glucose into cells from the bloodstream; **7** glucosuria and polyuria; **8** presence of glucose increases osmotic gradient of urine; **9** increased; **10** due to polyuria.

6.5.

Area	Hormone produced	Target	Action
Ovaries	Oestrogen (oestradiol)	Many systems	Prepares body for mating, e.g. swelling of vulva
	Progesterone (from corpus luteum)	Many systems	Maintains pregnancy
	Relaxin (from corpus luteum)	Muscles	Relaxes muscles prior to parturition
Testicles	Testosterone	Many systems	Secondary male characteristics
	Oestrogen	Many systems	Negative 'balance' to testosterone, i.e. feminization

6.6. **1** c; **2** a; **3** c; **4** b; **5** a; **6** d; **7** c; **8** b; **9** b; **10** b; **11** a; **12** c; **13** d; **14** a; **15** d; **16** d; **17** b; **18** c; **19** a; **20** b.

6.7.

V	A	S	O	P	R	E	S	S	I	N
	L	G							O	
	D	T	L						X	
N	O		H	U					Y	
I	S			Y	C				T	
T	T				R	A			O	
C	E					O	G		C	
A	R						X	O	I	
L	O		G	A	S	T	R	I	N	
O	N	R	E	L	A	X	I	N	N	
R	E									
P										

6.8. **1** false (this is the posterior pituitary); **2** true; **3** true; **4** false (the adrenal medulla produces adrenaline); **5** false (they produce insulin); **6** true; **7** false (the ovaries produce oestrogen); **8** true.

7 Heart and blood vascular system, lymphatic system, immune system

7.1. **1** Pulmonary arteries; **2** Aorta; **3** Pulmonary veins; **4** Left atrioventricular valve; **5** Chorda tendina; **6** Papillary muscle; **7** Interventricular septum; **8** Right atrioventricular valve; **9** Posterior vena cava; **10** Anterior vena cava.

7.2. The correct route is: vena cava; right atrium; right atrioventricular valve; right ventricle; pulmonary semilunar valve; pulmonary artery; lungs to be oxygenated; pulmonary vein; left atrium; left atrioventricular valve; left ventricle; aortic semilunar valve; aorta; around the body to distribute oxygen.

7.3. **1** myocardium; **2** Purkinje; **3** pacemaker; **4** bundle; **5** atria; **6** systole; **7** diastole; **8** fibrillation.

7.4. **1** 5–10; **2** 7.4; **3** haemoglobin; **4** oxygen; **5** transport; **6** hormones; **7** heat; **8** defence; **9** clotting; **10** albumin.

7.5. **1** Hypovolaemia—low circulating blood volume could be due to a number of factors, e.g. haemorrhage; **2** Hypoxia—poor oxygen saturation, could be due to a number of factors, e.g. respiratory disease; **3** Icterus (jaundice)—could be due to a number of factors, e.g. liver disease or abnormal erythrocyte breakdown; **4** Toxic shock, e.g. septicaemia; **5** Carbon monoxide poisoning.

7.6.

	L	E												I
	E		R		N			S			A			M
	U			Y	U		S	T			E			M
	C		S		T		L	L			R			U
	O		E		R	H	A	A	L	B	U	M	I	N
	C		T		I		R	S					W	O
	Y		Y		E		E	O					A	G
	T		C		N		N		C				T	L
	E		O		T		I			Y			E	O
	S		B		S		M				T		R	B
	E		M									E		U
	B	H	O	R	M	O	N	E	S				S	L
	U		R											I
	I		H											N
C	L	O	T	T	I	N	G	F	A	C	T	O	R	S

7.7. 7, 6, 3, 2, 5, 1, 4.

7.8. **1–8; 3–10; 5–2; 7–4; 9–6.**

7.9. 3, 4, 6, 2, 5, 1.

7.10. **1** Tunica media; **2** Tunica adventitia; **3** Artery; **4** Vein; **5** Tunica intima; **6** Capillary.

7.11. **1–10; 3–6; 5–2; 7–12; 9–4; 11–8.**

7.12. **1** thick walled; **2** thinner walled; **3** no; **4** yes; **5** deeper; **6** more superficial; **7** away from the heart; **8** towards the heart; **9** oxygenated; **10** deoxygenated.

7.13. **1** coronary arteries; **2** azygos vein; **3** coeliac artery; **4** aorta; **5** vena cava; **6** hepatic portal vein; **7** femoral artery; **8** brachial artery; **9** carotid artery; **10** cephalic vein.

7.14. **1** proteins; **2** interstitial; **3** protein; **4** fluid; **5** oedema; **6** fat; **7** small intestine; **8** lacteals; **9** bacteria; **10** macrophages; **11** lymphocytes; **12** antigens.

7.15. **1** more than blood vessels; **2** less than lymph vessels; **3** always carry lymph towards the heart; **4** carry blood both to and from the heart; **5** valves are present; **6** valves present in some (veins); **7** no smooth muscle; **8** smooth muscle.

7.16. Cisterna chyli/thoracic duct: left forelimb, thorax (left side), abdomen, right hindlimb, left hindlimb. Right lymphatic duct: head and neck, right forelimb, thorax (right side).

7.17. **1** Parotid lymph node; **2** Retropharyngeal lymph nodes; **3** Tracheal duct; **4** Thoracic duct; **5** Cisterna chyli; **6** Mesenteric lymph nodes; **7** Superficial inguinal lymph nodes; **8** Popliteal lymph node; **9** Bronchial lymph nodes; **10** Axillary lymph node; **11** Prescapular lymph node; **12** Submandibular lymph node.

7.18. **1** antibodies; **2** plasma cell; **3** virus; **4** antigen; **5** active; **6** vaccine; **7** passive; **8** antiserum; **9** colostrum.

7.19. **1** vena cava; **2** bicuspid or left atrioventricular valve; **3** cardiac septum; **4** left ventricle; **5** pulmonary artery; **6** ductus arteriosus; **7** apex; **8** epicardium; **9** sinuatrial node; **10** pulse.

7.20. **1** d; **2** a; **3** c; **4** b; **5** b; **6** a; **7** a; **8** a.

7.21. **1** c; **2** a; **3** c; **4** b; **5** d; **6** b; **7** d; **8** a; **9** b; **10** c.

7.22. **1** VENULE; **2** AZYGOS; **3** SERUM; **4** CORONARY ARTERY; **5** UREA; **6** LYMPHOCYTE; **7** AORTA; **8** RIGHT ATRIUM; **9** ANTIBODIES; **10** KIDNEY; **11** ERYTHROPOIESIS; **12** CLOT; **13** THROMBOCYTE; **14** SEPTUM.

7.23. **1** a; **2** a; **3** b; **4** d; **5** b.

7.24. **1** c; **2** b; **3** c; **4** c; **5** c.

8 The respiratory system

8.1. **1** gases; **2** oxygen; **3** carbon dioxide; **4** environment; **5** lungs; **6** body tissues; **7** bloodstream; **8** adenosine triphosphate; **9** carbon dioxide.

8.2. **1–10; 3–8; 5–16; 7–2; 9–6; 11–14; 13–4; 15–12.**

8.3. Epiglottis; arytenoids; interarytenoid; thyroid; crichoid.

8.4. **1** Larynx; **2** Annular ligaments; **3** Hyaline cartilage rings; **4** Right principal bronchus; **5** Left principal bronchus; **6** Bifurcation of the trachea.

8.5. **1** Bronchioles; **2** Principal bronchus; **3** Apical lobe; **4** Cardiac lobe; **5** Bronchi; **6** Alveolar duct; **7** Alveolus; **8** Hilus; **9** Accessory lobe.

8.6. Heart; trachea; lymphatic vessels; oesophagus; blood vessels; nerves.

8.7. **1** 79%; **2** 79%; **3** 21%; **4** 16%; **5** 0.04%; **6** 5%.

8.8. **1–6; 3–14; 5–2; 7–12; 9–4; 11–8; 13–10.**

8.9. Dog 10–30 breaths per minute. Cat 20–30 breaths per minute. Factors include activity level (sleeping, exercising, etc.), stress, pain, anaesthesia, pathology and oxygen content of air.

8.10. **1** b; **2** a; **3** c; **4** b; **5** b; **6** b; **7** d; **8** c; **9** d; **10** b; **11** a; **12** b; **13** c; **14** a; **15** c; **16** a; **17** d; **18** b.

8.11. **1** RESIDUAL VOLUME; **2** ETHMOID; **3** SEROUS; **4** PULMONARY; **5** INTERARYTENOID; **6** REFLEX; **7** ACCESSORY; **8** TURBINATE; **9** INHALATION; **10** OESOPHAGUS; **11** NARES.

9 The digestive system

9.1. **1** Zygomatic; **2** Sublingual; **3** Mandibular; **4** Parotid.

9.2. Prehension; lapping; manipulation of food; mechanical breakdown of food; panting; grooming.

9.3. **1** Crown; **2** Enamel; **3** Dentine; **4** Root; **5** Periodontal ligament; **6** Bone; **7** Pulp cavity; **8** Gum.

9.4. Tonsils; larynx; auditory canals; nasal cavity; oral cavity; tongue; oesophagus.

9.5. **1** Oesophagus; **2** Fundus; **3** Oesophageal (cardiac) sphincter; **4** Cardia; **5** Body; **6** Rugae; **7** Pyloric antrum; **8** Pyloric sphincter; **9** Duodenum.

9.6. Regurgitation is a passive process in which undigested food and/or fluid is returned from the stomach via the mouth shortly after eating or drinking. Vomiting is an active process in which food and/or liquid, which may or may not be partially digested, is returned from the gut tract via the mouth. It may or may not be shortly after eating.

9.7. **1** Lacteal; **2** Columnar epithelium; **3** Villus; **4** Crypt of Lieberkühn; **5** Goblet cell; **6** Brunner's gland; **7** Afferent blood supply; **8** Efferent blood supply.

9.8. 6; 13; 15; 2; 9; 1; 8; 17; 3; 11; 5; 10; 16; 7; 12; 14; 4.

9.9. Stomach: 30 seconds to 1 minute after swallowing. Small intestine: 2–4 hours. Rectum: 12–24 hours.

9.10. Pale: white meat; lack of bile pigment. Fatty: animal has eaten fat (e.g. block of butter); liver disease. Mucoid: colitis. Black: digested blood due to haemorrhage in the gastrointestinal tract; bloody meat eaten. Dry: constipation. Liquid: gastroenteritis.

9.11. **1** a; **2** d; **3** b; **4** b; **5** c; **6** b; **7** b; **8** c; **9** d; **10** c; **11** b; **12** b; **13** d; **14** c; **15** a; **16** a; **17** c; **18** c; **19** a; **20** c.

9.12. **1** FUNDUS; **2** INCISOR; **3** GASTR; **4** ENTER; **5** LIPASE; **6** FATTY ACIDS; **7** DISACCHARIDES; **8** ABDOMINAL; **9** DUODENUM; **10** ILEUM; **11** CARNASSIAL; **12** CARDIAC; **13** VOMITING; **14** DYSPHAGIA; **15** SMOOTH; **16** FAUCES; **17** TONSILS; **18** DESCENDING; **19** PYLORIC; **20** BACTERIA; **21** CRYPTS; **22** BOLUS.

9.13. Across: **1** BORBORYGMI; **2** SPHINCTER; **7** SUCROSE; **11** CAECUM; **12** FATS; **14** PTYALIN; **16** ILEUM; **17** DETOXIFICATION. Down: **1** BOLUS; **2** BICARBONATE; **3** RISES; **4** GUT; **6** COLIC; **8** UREA; **9** EFA; **10** AMMONIA; **13** PYLORIC; **14** PICA; **15** GRIND.

10 The urinary system

10.1. **1–12; 3–20; 5–14; 7–2; 9–16; 11–18; 13–8; 15–4; 17–10; 19–6.**

10.2. **1)** Complete; **1** Hilus, **2** Renal artery, **3** Renal vein, **4** Ureter; **2)** Sectioned; **5** Renal cortex-, **6** Renal pelvis, **7** Medulla, **8** Renal crest, **9** Calyces, **10** Renal capsule.

10.3. **1** Bowman's capsule; **2** Glomerulus; **3** Proximal convoluted tubule; **4** Distal convoluted tubule; **5** Collecting duct; **6** Descending loop of Henle; **7** Ascending loop of Henle; **8** Efferent arteriole; **9** Renal artery; **10** Afferent arteriole.

10.4. **1** glomerulus; **2** Bowman's; **3** ultrafiltrate; **4** proteins; **5** selective; **6** ECF; **7** urea; **8** collecting.

10.5. **1** Right kidney; **2** Renal artery and vein; **3** Left kidney; **4** Ureter; **5** Bladder; **6** Neck of bladder; **7** Urethra.

10.6. **1** straw; **2** straw; **3** nil to mild, male urine may smell stronger; **4** nil to mild, male urine may smell stronger; **5** clear liquid; **6** clear liquid; **7** 5.2–6.8; **8** 6–7; **9** 1.015–1.045; **10** 1.020–1.040; **11** 1–2; **12** 1–2.

10.7. **1** c; **2** c; **3** d; **4** c; **5** b; **6** b; **7** d; **8** c; **9** b; **10** c.

10.8.

M	I	C	T	U	R	I	T	I	O	N
		R		R						E
	S	E	L	E	C	T	I	V	E	P
		S	N	T		B		I		H
		T	I	E		R		T		R
N			N	R		O		A		I
E			E			S		M	E	T
P		U	R	E	A	B		I	L	I
H						A		N	U	S
R						E		D	B	
O	G	L	O	M	E	R	U	L	U	S
N									T	

11 The reproductive system

11.1. **1–6**; **3–10**; **5–2**; **7–4**; **9–12**; **11–8**.

11.2. **1** Tunica vaginalis; **2** Efferent tubules; **3** Septa; **4** Seminiferous tubules; **5** Epididymis; **6** Spermatic cord.

11.3. **1** 40 days; **2** at birth.

11.4. **1** Corpus cavernosum; **2** Bulbus glandis; **3** Retractor penis; **4** Corpus spongiosum; **5** Urethra; **6** Os penis.

11.5. **1** Fold of peritoneum becoming mesovarium; **2** Ovarian (suspensory) ligament; **3** Ovary; **4** Ovarian bursa.

11.6. **1** 2–27 days; **2** FSH, LH, oestrogen later; **3** extremely swollen vulva, bloody vaginal discharge, teases male; **4** 3–21 days; **5** LH, oestrogen, progesterone after ovulation; **6** soft but swollen vulva, straw-coloured vaginal discharge, will accept male; **7** 30–90 days; **8** progesterone, prolactin; **9** vulval swelling and discharge slowly diminish pseudopregnancy later; **10** approx. 4 months; **11** period of quiescence; **12** normal appearance and behaviour.

11.7. 4; 6; 9; 5; 3; 7; 2; 8; 1.

11.8. **1** a; **2** c; **3** a; **4** c; **5** b; **6** a; **7** c; **8** d.

11.9. **1** ventral, between the hindlegs; **2** caudal, beneath the anus; **3** sparse; **4** good hair covering; **5** absent; **6** present; **7** ventral, pointing cranially; **8** caudal, pointing caudally; **9** bony os penis present; **10** no bone present; **11** smooth; **12** barbed; **13** long and curved; **14** shorter and straighter.

11.10. **1** Prostate gland; **2** Testicle; **3** Penis; **4** Deferent duct; **5** Epididymis; **6** Bladder.

11.11. **1** a, **2** c, **3** b, **4** c, **5** d, **6** d, **7** b, **8** c, **9** a, **10** a, **11** b, **12** c, **13** b, **14** b, **15** a.

11.12. **1** Oviduct; **2** Infundibulum; **3** Vestibule; **4** Vulva; **5** Clitoris; **6** External urethral orifice; **7** Vagina; **8** Uterine body; **9** Urinary bladder; **10** Uterine horn; **11** Ovary.

12 The skin and hair

12.1. **1** bacteria; **2** sebum; **3** keratin; **4** camouflage; **5** pacinian; **6** vibrissae; **7** pheromones; **8** sudoriferous; **9** digital; **10** ergosterol; **11** arrector; **12** vasoconstriction; **13** vasodilation; **14** panting.

12.2. **1** Epidermis; **2** Dermis; **3** Hypodermis; **4** Hair follicle; **5** Sensory receptor; **6** Sudoriferous gland; **7** Arrector pili muscle; **8** Sebaceous gland; **9** Dermal papillae.

12.3. **1** Teat orifice; **2** Teat canal; **3** Teat sinus; **4** Gland sinus; **5** Lobules of glandular tissue; **6** Connective tissue.

12.4. **1** b; **2** b; **3** b; **4** c; **5** a; **6** d; **7** c; **8** c; **9** a; **10** d; **11** b; **12** b; **13** b; **14** d; **15** a.

13 Birds

13.1. **1** Alula (first digit); **2** Major metacarpal; **3** Second digit; **4** Ulna; **5** Radius; **6** Thoracic vertebrae; **7** Uncinate process; **8** Synsacrum; **9** Coccygeal vertebrae; **10** Pygostyle; **11** Ischium; **12** Pubis; **13** Femur; **14** Tarsometatarsus; **15** Hallux; **16** Tibiotarsus; **17** Complete rib; **18** Sternum; **19** Coracoid; **20** Cervical vertebrae; **21** Lower mandible; **22** Upper mandible; **23** Orbit; **24** Scapula; **25** Humerus

13.2. **1** Oesophagus; **2** Crop; **3** Proventriculus; **4** Ventriculus (gizzard); **5** Caecum/caecae; **6** Cloaca; **7** Intestine; **8** Pancreatic ducts; **9** Pancreas; **10** Bile ducts; **11** Spleen; **12** Liver

13.3. **1** c; **2** d; **3** b; **4** d; **5** a

14 Exotic mammals

14.1. **1** b; **2** b; **3** d; **4** a; **5** d

15 Reptiles

15.1. **1** c; **2** c; **3** b; **4** c; **5** c; **6** a

16 The horse

16.1. **1** Cervical vertebrae; **2** Thoracic vertebrae; **3** Lumbar vertebrae; **4** Sacrum; **5** Coccygeal vertebrae; **6** Femur; **7** Fibula; **8** Tibia; **9** Tarsal bones; **10** Metatarsal bones; **11** Proximal phalanx hindlimb; **12** Middle phalanx hindlimb; **13** Distal phalanx hindlimb; **14** Patella; **15** Pelvis; **16** Rib; **17** Sternum; **18** Accessory carpal bone; **19** Proximal sesamoid; **20** Distal sesamoid; **21** Distal phalanx forelimb; **22** Middle phalanx forelimb; **23** Proximal phalanx forelimb; **24** Metacarpus; **25** Carpus; **26** Radius; **27** Ulna; **28** Humerus; **29** Scapula; **30** Skull

16.2. C7 T18 L6 S5 Cd15–20

16.3. **1** Knee; **2** Cannon bone; **3** Splint bones; **4** Long pastern; **5** Short pastern; **6** Pedal bone; **7** Fetlock joint; **8** Navicular bone; **9** Coffin joint; **10** Pastern joint

16.4. **1** Proximal sesamoid bone; **2** Superficial digital flexor tendon; **3** Sesamoidian ligaments; **4** Deep digital flexor tendon; **5** Distal sesamoid (navicular bone); **6** Digital cushion; **7** White line; **8** Hoof wall; **9** Extensor tendon; **10** Metacarpal III; **11** Water line; **12** White line; **13** Point of frog; **14** Frog; **15** Sole; **16** Bars; **17** Seat of corn (angle of heel); **18** Buttress of heel; **19** Commissures; **20** Cleft or frog; **21** Bulbs; **22** Heel; **23** Quarters; **24** Toe

16.5. **1** cornea; **2** choroid; **3** tapetum lucidum; **4** optic disc; **5** ciliary; **6** lens; **7** retina; **8** iris; **9** corpora nigra; **10** light; **11** ramp; **12** muscle

16.6. **1** VI; **2** V; **3** IV; **4** III; **5** II; **6** I; **7** Di3; **8** I2; **9** I1; **10** I1; **11** I2; **12** I3; **13** C1; **14** Diastema; **15** P1; **16** P2; **17** P3; **18** P4; **19** M1; **20** M2; **21** M3

16.7. **1** long-day breeder; **2** Spring; **3** Summer; **4** seasonally polyoestrous; **5** spontaneous ovulator; **6** 17–21; **7** on heat; **8** 3–5; **9** Ovulation; **10** 14–16; **11** Oestrus; **12** anoestrous

16.8. **1** c; **2** a; **3** b; **4** a; **5** b; **6** b

References and further reading

Aspinall V (Ed) 2006 The Complete Textbook of Veterinary Nursing. Butterworth Heinemann, Edinburgh

Aspinall V, Capello M 2009 Introduction to Veterinary Anatomy and Physiology Textbook, 2nd edn. Butterworth Heinemann, Edinburgh

Aspinall V, O'Reilly M 2004 Introduction to Veterinary Anatomy and Physiology. Butterworth Heinemann, Edinburgh

Bowden C, Masters J 2001 Pre-veterinary Nursing Textbook. Butterworth Heinemann/BVNA, Edinburgh

Blood D C, Studdert V P 2007 Saunders' Comprehensive Veterinary Dictionary, 3rd edn. Saunders, Edinburgh

Boyd J S 2001 Colour Atlas of Clinical Anatomy of the Dog and Cat, 2nd edn. Mosby, St Louis

College of Animal Welfare 2000 300 Questions & Answers in Anatomy and Physiology. Butterworth Heinemann, Edinburgh

College of Animal Welfare 2003 300 Questions & Answers in Medical and General Nursing for Veterinary Nurses. Butterworth Heinemann, Edinburgh

College of Animal Welfare, Tartaglia L, Waugh A 2005 Veterinary Physiology and Applied Anatomy – Revised Reprint: A Textbook for Veterinary Nurses and Technicians. Butterworth Heinemann/BSAVA, Edinburgh

Colville T P, Bassert J M 2002 Clinical Anatomy and Physiology for Veterinary Technicians. Mosby, St Louis

Colville T P, Bassert J M 2008 Clinical Anatomy and Physiology for Veterinary Technicians, 2nd edn. Mosby, St Louis

Dyce KM, Sack WO, Wensing JG 2002 Textbook of Veterinary Anatomy, 3rd edn. Saunders, St Louis

Evans H 1993 Miller's Anatomy of the Dog, 3rd edn. Saunders, Philadelphia

Gosden C (Ed) 2004 Exotics and Wildlife: A Manual of Veterinary Nursing Care. Butterworth Heinemann, Edinburgh

Hine R 1988 Concise Veterinary Dictionary. Oxford University Press, Oxford

Lane D, Cooper B 1999 Veterinary Nursing, 2nd edn. Butterworth Heinemann/BSAVA, Edinburgh

Lane D, Cooper B 2007 Veterinary Nursing, 4th edn. BSAVA

Lane DR, Guthrie S, Griffith S 2007 Dictionary of Veterinary Nursing. Butterworth Heinemann, Oxford

Masters J, Martin C 2007 Animal Nursing Assistant Textbook. Butterworth Heinemann/Elsevier, Philadelphia

McBride DF 2001 Learning Veterinary Terminology, 2nd edn. Elsevier, USA

Reece W 1997 The Physiology of Domestic Animals, 2nd edn. Williams & Wilkins, Baltimore

Printed in the United States
By Bookmasters